For You

Andreas Seidl

Handover of Power

Global Version

Volume 15: Health

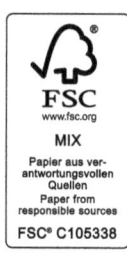

Imprint

Bibliographic information of the German National Library:
The German National Library lists this publication in the
German National Bibliography; detailed bibliographic data
are available on the Internet at http://dnb.dnb.de.

© 2022 Dipl. Pol. Theodor Andreas Seidl

Cover: Christiane Ebrecht
Translation: DeepL, Cologne
Production and publishing: BoD – Books on Demand,
Norderstedt

ISBN: 978-3-7562-0256-0

Acknowledgements

My thanks go to my family and friends who have made me who I am today. Special thanks to all those who supported me in writing this book. I would like to thank all my classmates, teachers, fellow students, lecturers, demonstrators, activists, colleagues, companies and countries with whom I have had the privilege of sharing the experiences from which all the ideas in this book have emerged. I would like to thank the staff of Books on Demand for their kind helpfulness. I thank the citizens of Seligenstadt for the harmony and solidarity in which I was able to write.

Foreword

This policy concept contains a variety of proposals for possible political reforms. It can be peacefully and democratically adapted to any current political system of any state in the world, but also to political systems in families, clubs, associations or companies. Wherever humans make or submit to rules that manage living together, the following proposals can be helpful. Readers who find the proposals so helpful that they would like to implement them together with like-minded people can contact the author. The contact form on the last page can be used for this purpose.

Faults and defects

I ask for your understanding that this volume was not professionally proofread. I could only afford professional proofreading for the summary. Spelling errors and unfortunate phrasing may therefore occur. As soon as this volume has sold enough to pay for a professional proofreading, it will be done. After that, a new edition will be published.

English version

Please understand that this volume has been translated automatically. I could only afford a professional translation for the summary. Poor wording and spelling errors may therefore occur. In case of doubt, the German version shall prevail. As soon as this volume has sold enough to pay for a professional translation, it will be done. After that, a new edition will be published. It was more important to me that no one in the world should have an information advantage than individual translation errors in the complete work.

References

If something has been quoted directly, it is set in italics. If the headings contain footnotes, the sources for direct and indirect quotations apply in the chapter for which the heading stands. Otherwise, quotations or source references are directly at the word or at the end of the sentence or paragraph. This book contains parts of text based on the Federal Constitution of the Swiss Confederation of 18 April 1999 (as of 12 February 2017), abbreviated to BV[1] and the Constitution of the Canton of Bern of 6 June 1993 (as of 11 March 2015), abbreviated to KV[2].

If the constitutional paragraph, or individual paragraphs thereof, are based in whole or in part on extracts from the BV or KV, this is indicated in a footnote. The references to the corresponding footnotes for constitutional paragraphs are usually found after the heading of the affected chapter and sometimes in the body of the text. Articles used in the Swiss constitutions are listed in the footnote with a number after the title of the constitutional paragraph. Example: §123 Sample title: BV Art.123, KV Art.123.

All internet sources are fully cited in the footnotes. They were last accessed on 30.09.2021. All literature sources are also listed in full in the footnotes.

All references to tasks undertaken by other ministries and described in more detail there are given in footnotes. Example: Model Ministry - 1.2.3 Model Chapter.

All footnotes are to be viewed in comparison to the respective source, so-called indirect quotations. Direct quotations are set in italics, but hardly ever occur. The source reference is intended to enable further investigation and to take copyright

---

1 This is not an official publication. Only the publication by the Swiss Federal Chancellery is authoritative. https://www.fedlex.admin.ch/eli/cc/1999/404/de On 14.12.2021

2 This is not an official publication. The Bernese Official Collection of Laws is authoritative. https://www.belex.sites.be.ch/frontend/versions/2420?locale=de#ART71 On 16.12.2021

into account.

Table of contents

1 Goals of the Ministry of Health

The Ministry of Health aims to keep the population as healthy as possible, to enable them to live a long life and to maintain or improve the existing environmental conditions for future generations.

Basically, the health of humans, nature and the planetary ecosystem should be seen as a unity that can be mutually dependent. Therefore, this ministry is concerned with keeping humans and the environment healthy.

Basically, every body belongs to the human being personally. He has the right to make it sick, poison it or keep it untrained, as long as he does not endanger the health of others. The Ministry of Health pursues a policy of ensuring the healthiest possible conditions in the citizens' environment.

The individual goals include the prevention, containment and eradication of diseases and toxins. To this end, all citizens should have access to a healthcare system that is capable of continuously monitoring the effectiveness of treatment and care and improving it through research. The aim is to link the collected data as well as possible so that diagnoses can be related to treatment methods and environmental conditions.

The aim of health care is to keep patient records in such a way that physicians can coordinate their treatments with the patient's health pathway and with their treating colleagues. This also pursues the goal of avoiding interactions between medicines and drugs.

Vices are expressly permitted to humans and they should be given the opportunity to care for them as healthily as possible. The Ministry of Health aims to make drugs as pure as possible, to enable preventive measures against addiction and to protect bystanders from the damage to health caused by addictive substances. Another goal is to design health insurance schemes in such a way that insured persons can separate their general and special personal needs.

What humans are explicitly not allowed to do is pollute the environment. The aim is to prevent future generations from having to grow up in a poisoned, polluted environment that is hostile to humans and distant from nature and, in the worst case, from dying out because of it. With its requirements, the Ministry of Health is pursuing the goal of increasingly improving conditions for future generations through technical and social progress. The aim is to achieve the most complete possible understanding of the health of human bodies and that of all organisms on earth, thus making it possible for humans to design stable ecosystems. In this way, the Ministry of Health is conducting the basic research needed to relocate ecosystems that can maintain their own health to other planets. The long-term goal of the Ministry of Health is that humanity does not become extinct and survives the galactically willed end of the Earth on other planets with its natural environment.

2 Departments

The departments are divided into sub-departments and enumerations are usually considered as their individual units. Many tasks of some departments are completely taken over by other ministries as a service.

2.1 Central Department

Part of the Central Department is the Reception Office with the Courier and Mail Room, which directs all concerns, broadcasts and visitors to the appropriate place in the ministry.

2.1.1 Staff

The Human Resources Department is responsible for staff development and planning. For this purpose, it takes care of the recruitment of junior staff, intern and trainee programmes as well as the selection procedures for employees and special selection procedures for applicants with disabilities. For politicians and employees, the department prepares a job plan. In all its tasks, it works in voting with the personnel board.[1]
All other personnel matters are transferred to the respective ministries. The Ministry of Education is responsible for the training and further education of employees for the state

---

1 Ministry of State Organisation - 2.1.1.1 Personnel board

service.[2] The Ministry of Labour takes over the service law.[3] This includes the labour and collective bargaining law of employees in the state service, remuneration, personnel administration of all careers and employees, flexitime, holiday and sick leave, working time with or without flexitime in part-time or full-time at the place of work or in home work. The Ministry of Infrastructure provides housing assistance for all state employees.[4] The Ministry of Finance's Pay Office takes care of employees' salary, expenses, travel and relocation costs.[5] The Ministry of Education provides childcare for all employees in the state service.[6]

2.1.1.1 Company medical service

The company medical service ensures that occupational health management is carried out for all workplaces in the state service in order to prevent service accidents and occupational diseases. The health auditors of the Company Auditing Agency[7] carry out the corresponding audits on a regular basis. However, if occupational accidents and diseases do occur, affected workers are entitled to free occupational health and safety protection. Treatment is provided in state hospitals and university clinics. The occupational health service provides legal and technical supervision of the treatment provided and carries out pre-employment examinations, health tests and vaccinations whenever such examinations are required.

Employees of the ministries of security and foreigners who are returnees from crisis areas receive psychological care. For this purpose, there is a contact point and psychological care for employees who are returnees from crisis areas, their families or partners.

---

2 Ministry of Education - 2.1.1.1 Education and training for the state service
3 Ministry of Labour - 4 State enterprises, 13 Labour Directory
4 Ministry of Infrastructure - 2.1.1.1 Housing assistance for state service employees
5 Ministry of Finance - 2.1.1.1 Staff remuneration
6 Ministry of Education - 2.1.1.2 Childcare for state service employees
7 Ministry of Labor - 20 Company Auditing Agency

2.1.2 Organisation

The ministries of media, security, justice, finance, labour, state organisation provide audit services for quality management in the ministry, evaluation of work performance, revenues and expenditures, as well as corruption prevention, sabotage protection and, if necessary, disciplinary matters.[8]

The Ministry of Labour regulates procurement law and ensures corruption-free state orders and procurement.[9] The Ministry of Finance organises the annual budget vote and ensures proper accounting in each ministry.[10] It regulates budget procedures, budget law, staff budgets, departmental budgets, costs and cash management, and assists ministries in budget planning for the budget vote. The language service for translating talks or texts is provided by the Ministry of Education.[11]

The Ministry of Digital Affairs supports the supply of Information Technology.[12] In voting with the Procurement Office of the Ministry of Labour, it takes care of the procurement, provision, maintenance and service of technical devices and software. Much of this is produced in-house to ensure data protection in information and communication technology. Information technology and digitalisation officers audit and advise the ministries. Digital appointment calendar and documentation services are provided as well as a digital policy archive including a library.

2.2 Management Department

The Management Department is the minister's department. With his office team, he provides policy planning and analysis for his ministry and coordinates the relationship between the nation and the municipality through exchanges with his deputies in the municipalities. He initiates cooperation with

8 Ministries of Media, Security, Justice, Finance, State Organisation - 2.1.2.1 Audit services
9 Ministry of Labour - 6 Procurement Office
10 Ministry of Finance - 8 state revenues, 9 state expenditure
11 Ministry of Education - 2.1.3 Language Service
12 Ministry of Digital Affairs - 2.1.2.1.1 Supply of Information Technology

other ministries or citizens in committees and is supported by the Ministry of State Organisation.

The Ministry of Media Affairs, through its media service, provides press and public relations for the ministry, moderates civil dialogue, trains or provides a spokesperson for the minister, writes speeches and texts on request, and ensures the implementation of conferences and events.[13]

The Ministry of Digital Affairs is responsible for digital management and thus provides departmental management. It automatically produces business statistics, staff surveys and the current state of research through statistics. It automatically forwards proposals to the affected or empowered state employees. In document management, it ensures digitalisation and that ministries share forms with each other.[14]

2.3 Foreign Department

The Foreign Department ensures compliance with the requirements of the G7 and G20 conventions, international law, international trade law, the United Nations Agenda 2030 with its 17 Sustainable Development Goals (SDGs)[15] and cooperation with the OECD. If the international requirements are weaker, the stricter domestic requirements are binding inland. If the requirements impede domestic health policy, the people decide whether international treaties should be respected, terminated or renegotiated.

Because diseases, air and water pollution know no national borders, as many international agreements as possible are being reached to keep humanity as healthy as possible. International food safety policy, the health status of animals and plants for export, water protection law and environmental protection policy are being standardised.

---

13 Ministry of Media Affairs - 2.2.1.1 Media Service
14 Ministry of Digital Affairs - 2.1.2.1 Digital Service
15 https://www.bundesregierung.de/breg-de/themen/
nachhaltigkeitspolitik/nachhaltigkeitsziele-verstaendlich-erklaert-232174

2.4 Health Care Department

The Health Care Department oversees each Health Committee and ensures cooperation with other ministries during an extraordinary situation. It ensures the operation of the Health Card, Health Directory[16] and Care Directory in cooperation with the Ministry of Digital Affairs. Together with the Minister of Health, it develops the draft laws for the conditions and procedures for the licensing of physicians and their duties. Together with the Medical Association, it ensures the negotiation of treatments and prices in the Medical Fee Schedule. It operates the health centres in cooperation with the Ministry of Planned Economy and the university hospitals with the Ministry of Education. It conducts negotiations on quantities and prices with the Pharmaceutical Industry Association. With the Minister of Health, it drafts legislation on the purity law and on the dispensing and research of drugs. It operates the General Health Insurance as well as the Addictive drugs Health Insurance and Immortality Health Insurance. It votes between the ministries of economy on the insurance services in the economic forms. It agrees with the Association of Health Insurance Funds on delimitations for the obligations of health insurance funds to cover health care costs.

2.5 Health Prevention Department

The Health Prevention Department oversees the health agencies, health auditors and institutes of the Ministry of Health. It operates the Environment Directory in cooperation with the Ministry of Digital Affairs. It issues recommendations on nutrition and exercise to citizens, working with the ministries of education and media. It ensures the implementation of food and product safety standards in cooperation with the Ministry of Labour. Together with the ministries of labour and economy, it ensures the implementation of the circular economy and sustainable use of nature. Together with the Minister of Health, it develops draft legislation on the

---

16Ministry of Digital - 12 Directories

sustainable use of nature, environmental protection and structural change. In cooperation with the ministries of labour and infrastructure, it ensures the implementation of measures to protect the environment and raw materials.

3 Tasks of the Ministry of Health

The Ministry of Health's task is to support sufficient and advanced care and prevention for the health of humans and the environment. The ministry in the capital city prepares laws that form the basis for requirements and measures. The Health Agencies are responsible for publishing the requirements and implementing regulations for measures. They inform affected citizens as quickly as possible and comprehensively as necessary. Company Auditing Agency health auditors check compliance with the requirements and the proper execution of the measures.

Through the healthcare system, health prevention and health care are linked and contribute to the maintenance of health and rapid recovery of humans and the environment. The link is established through the health, care and environmental directories and the citizen is involved as a patient, caregiver or environmental protector. Diagnoses can be related to treatment methods and environmental conditions through the link. The task of the Ministry of Health is to distinguish ineffective from effective treatment methods or environmental protection policies, to prevent ineffective ones and to develop effective ones.

Through its institutes, the Ministry of Health brings the necessary expertise to justify the decisions for requirements and measures to the population. Through the equalisation of the medical appeal as a "physician", a wide variety of healing methods and remedies are applied, tested, further developed and put into relation and interaction with each other. By legalising drugs and other addictive substances, the Ministry of Health achieves an opportunity for addiction prevention, appropriate personal dosage and the protection of third parties from the use of addictive substances.

The Ministry of Health enables the individual, through the election of health insurance, to satisfy his or her personal needs to use addictive substances that are harmful to health or to live as long as possible, as he or she sees fit, without having to charge the costs of this to other insured persons for general health care.

The Ministry of Health is responsible for protecting consumers and the environment. The task is fulfilled through proposals and requirements for healthy nutrition and exercise as well as safety requirements for food, products and sustainable use of nature. The institutes provide the necessary measurement and research. Company Auditing Agency auditors ensure the awarding of test and quality seals for goods and services, the licensing of personnel, medical products and institutions in the health sector, the measurement of the exposure of the environment to toxic and hazardous substances, and the introduction of innovations to prevent exposure in the future.

4 Healthcare system[17]

The Ministry of Health regulates the necessary requirements about the healthcare system in the following health law. The healthcare system ensures the holistic health of the population. Holistic here means the care of illnesses and injuries as well as the maintenance of health through healthy nutrition, exercise, products and environmental conditions.

Health care is provided by physicians and physician assistants in practices and hospitals. They provide medical and nursing care for sick or impaired patients. Pharmacists and the pharmaceutical industry support patients and physicians with the necessary medicines. Accidents become rarer due to requirements in occupational and product safety, and diseases are eradicated through vaccinations or treated according to the latest research. Health insurance companies and the Medical Fee Schedule support economic care.

Health safety is monitored by the Health Agency and is guaranteed when both the population is supported by a sufficient number of medical practices and hospitals and the

---

17§236,1 Public health: KV Art.41, §237,1 Protection of health and environment: BV Art. 118

standards for the protection of humans and nature are met by companies and private individuals. The standards are derived from research and measurement results of the institutes of the Ministry of Health.

4.1 Health Agency[18]

The Health Agency is responsible for cooperation between the authorities and institutions of the Ministry of Health and with other ministries, their institutions and companies. It audits all requirements in the healthcare system that are not audited by the Company Auditing Agency. It instructs the health auditors in new requirements and carries out spot checks on the work of the health auditors, undercover if necessary. It has its headquarters in the capital city of the Ministry of Health and branches in all town halls.

The Health Agency is particularly important when it comes to controlling or eliminating communicable, common or deadly diseases. This applies to humans as well as to animals and plants. In order to contain and eradicate communicable diseases, it can force the pharmaceutical industry to do a certain amount of vaccine research for a limited period of time. It must then work with the Ministry of Education to provide a research network[19] for these research projects. Common diseases are reduced through preventive measures such as a healthy diet and sufficient exercise. Common diseases due to an addictive drug will be included in research on the purity law and funded through the Addictive drugs Health Insurance. Research is conducted on fatal diseases. The Health Agency initiates research in the Research Directory[20] and funds it through the Immortality Health Insurance.

The Health Agency is responsible for determining whether a living being is conscious and classifies it accordingly. Consciousness is the sensory perception of a stimulus as well as the subsequent planned, purposeful and thought-out reaction, in connection with a memory, sensation of pain and

18 §237.2b Protection of health and the environment: BV Art. 118
19 Ministry of Education - 4.10.4 Research Network
20 Ministry of Innovation - 5.3 Research Directory

happiness.

The Health Agency monitors the confidentiality of the Health Directory data and the equitable division of subject areas for physicians, physician assistants, nurses and pharmacists. To do this, it works with the associations for physicians, pharmacists and the pharmaceutical industry. It sets capacity limits for health care institutions. It agrees with the retail sector on the dispensing of drugs, what requirements apply and how they can be implemented.

4.2 Extraordinary situation

The Ministry of Health has special responsibilities in an exceptional situation with a high risk to the health of the entire population. If possible, it shall enact an appropriate health protection law in times without such an extraordinary situation. This law lays down measures to protect against infection with pathogens or the absorption of toxic contaminants into the body. This law is capable of restricting the fundamental constitutional rights of citizens. This is justified by the principle of protecting the health safety of all inhabitants of the country by restricting the freedom of individuals. The people must be able to negotiate the measures in a committee[21] and vote on them individually in a referendum. The people thereby determine what ratio of freedom and security they want in the extraordinary situation. If those entitled to vote in an individual municipality want to accept harsher measures by a majority, they can enact them as municipal laws without having to hold a subsidiarity vote in advance. These municipal laws are always limited to the duration of the extraordinary situation. During the extraordinary situation, the state of exception applies if it occurs suddenly and measures become necessary that have not been regulated in laws so far.[22] Laws declared as urgent without a constitutional basis can apply immediately in the extraordinary situation and must be submitted to the people for voting within 14 days. The veto quorum[23] applies from the

21 Ministry of State Organisation - 9.6 Committee
22 Ministry of State Organisation - 12.6 State of exception
23 Ministry of State Organisation - 9.5.14 Veto quorum

start of the legislative process and also applies to regulations that are intended to provisionally replace the missing law. The veto quorum can be triggered for all regulations concerning the handling of the special situation or for each individual regulation. If the veto quorum is supported by 50% of the population, all regulations affected must be immediately repealed and the corresponding legislative process must be held in committee.

The Health Agency is responsible for involving the appropriate institute in the measurement, forecasting and planning of appropriate measures and, if necessary, for running the healthcare system on a Planned Economy basis for the duration of the emergency. The Minister of Health is responsible for this Planned Economy government and is assisted by the Minister of Planned Economy and all necessary ministries in the fulfilment of his tasks during the extraordinary situation.

4.3 Health committee[24]

The Minister of Health must convene a committee for all laws that may affect the dignity and personality of a person. He can decide whether only affected citizens are involved or the people. The people can convene or participate in a committee at any time through the veto quorum and the repeal quorum.[25] Laws that affect the dignity of humans and their personality are research projects on humans that are to be carried out on persons who are not capable of judgement. This also applies to human inheritance and germinal material. Freedom of research may only be restricted if the health of society could be endangered or if research is to be carried out on individuals against their will. The same applies to artificial intelligence and machines capable of judgement that acquire consciousness. The party wings of the health party can convene an ethics commission[26] for existing conditions, laws or ongoing legislative processes. Citizens can use a veto quorum to apply

24 §239.1 Research on humans: BV Art. 118b, §240,2 Reproductive medicine and gene technology in the human field: BV Art. 119
25 Ministry of State Organisation - 9.6 Committee, 9.5.14 Veto quorum, 9.5.15 Repeal quorum
26 Ministry of State Organisation - 8.5.9 Ethics Commission

the ethics committee procedure in a committee.

The Health Committee is also convened when the Medical Fee Schedule is rejected in the budget vote. In individual cases, it is also used for the negotiation of contentious laws.

4.4 Company Auditing Agency health auditor[27]

The Company Auditing Agency's health auditors are expert employees of the ministries of health and education who perform their service in the Company Auditing Agency on a rotational basis. Namely, they are physicians, teachers in the subject areas of medicine, biology, chemistry, geology and environmental sciences. They work at the place of employment where the areas, companies or ministries to be examined are located. The Institutes of Occupational and Environmental Medicine are located in the capital city of the Ministry of Health.

The health auditors ensure compliance with the requirements for occupational safety and environmental protection[28] and are supported in this by the institutes for occupational safety and environmental protection. If hazards are identified, the health auditors document them and forward them to appropriate research institutions. They arrange for a study to be conducted to determine the extent of the hazard and to develop innovations to eliminate the hazard. The cost of these services is borne by the companies that caused the hazard. If requirements are necessary, the health auditors propose legislation to the Minister of Health.

4.4.1 Damage limitation[29]

The health and technology auditors test products and production methods for harmful substances and determine the costs of disposal in cooperation with the economic auditors.

---

27 §189.3 Sustainability: BV Art. 73
28 Ministry of Labour - 14.2 Occupational safety and health, 14.3 Environmental protection
29 §190,4,7 Environmental protection: KV Art.31, 36, BV Art.74, §239,2d,2e Research on humans: BV Art. 118b, §240,1 Reproductive

The results are used to calculate the price surcharge on the products that must be paid to the disposal companies.

The innovation auditors notify the health auditors if biological or medical research projects are to be examined. The health auditors check whether persons who are to be involved in the research are adequately protected. They check this newly at the regular review meetings, as well as the rest of the laws on health protection in biological and medical research.

In particular, the health auditors examine and investigate suspected abuses in reproductive medicine and genetic engineering. If they find abuses, violations or deficiencies, they identify which goods need to be seized to eliminate the abuse and cooperate with the police in the preliminary investigation.

To calculate the amount of tariffs on goods and services that pose a risk to environmental or health protection, the health auditors examine the products and calculate the costs of releasing pollutants during their use and disposal. If they have concerns about the dubiousness of products to be imported, they propose a general import ban to the Minister of Health and a specific import ban to the Health Agency for the affected shipment.

4.4.2 Health risks[30]

The health auditors ensure the highest possible quality in health care by auditing state and private health care facilities, the pharmaceutical industry and its products, as well as the licensing of physicians, physician assistants and pharmacists. Violations that are not remedied in a timely manner result in a temporary or indefinite operating or occupational ban.

When genetic engineering is used in the human sector and in agriculture[31] , the applicable requirements are monitored, deficiencies are noted in the test report, deadlines are set for rectification and violations are reported to the legality auditors.

medicine and genetic engineering in the human field: BV Art. 119, §152,2 Tariffs
30 §222,1,2,6 Money games: BV Art.106, §236,4 Health care: KV Art.41, §239,2d,2e Research on humans: BV Art. 118b
31 Ministry of Labour - 19.8.1 Animal products, 19.8.2 Plant products

The health auditors check companies in which addictive drugs are consumed to see whether all consumers are sufficiently protected and pay into the Addictive drugs Health Insurance appropriately. In the case of money games in particular, they check whether operations are manipulated, how high the distributed profits are to owners and players, and whether information on addiction prevention has reached players. New types and locations for money games or intoxicants must be checked by health auditors for their addictive effect and the expected loss of health or money before they are introduced to the market.

4.4.3 Drinking water and forests[32]

The health auditors are responsible for the regular inspection of pipes, sources and storage facilities of drinking water. If contamination is found, the health auditors may order the affected Municipal Utilities Company[33] to remove the contamination in due time and temporarily shut down the affected drinking water supply. For this purpose, the Health Agency may sue companies and private individuals who are proven to be responsible for the contamination for damages and prohibit the polluting acts or the use of the affected area. The health auditors receive guideline values from the Institute of Environmental Medicine on what condition forests must have in order to maintain their protective and welfare functions. For this purpose, samples are taken from the soil, the trees and the air and evaluated. If the protective and welfare functions of the forest are impaired in cities or forest areas, the health auditors may authorise the Ministry of Infrastructure to manage the forest on its own responsibility for a limited period of time and to charge the owner for their services.

---

32 §192.7 Water, §193.1 Forest: BV Art. 77
33 Ministry of Infrastructure - 4.9 Municipal Utilities Company

4.5 Institutes of the Ministry of Health[34]

The institutes of the Ministry of Health are responsible for identifying which diseases, goods and services endanger environmental or health protection. They make proposals on how to avoid the hazard through research and development or regulations and how to design a sustainable use of nature. This includes in particular how the environment can be protected in such a way that it can also keep future generations of humans, animals and plants healthy.

4.5.1 Institute for Medicines and Food

The Institute for Medicines and Food investigates adverse effects of medicines, medical devices, food and other goods that are to be imported into the human body. It tests the products before they are launched on the market and in long-term studies.

If adverse effects are detected, this is communicated to the affected companies and the health auditors. If adverse effects continue to be measured, the Institute proposes a ban or regularisation of the affected product to the Minister of Health.

4.5.2 Institute for Diseases and Vaccines

The Institute for Diseases and Vaccines collects all known diseases worldwide and links them to appropriate treatments, medicines and vaccines and registers them in a database in the Health Directory. It compiles appropriate protective measures against infectious diseases and coordinates research into protective measures and vaccines by private and state research institutions.

The Institute is able to connect various research-based pharmaceutical companies and colleges or institutes into a research and industrial community through the Company Auditing Agency's data transfer, if through cooperation infections can be detected more quickly or vaccines can be

34 §189.3 Sustainability, §236.5c Health, §152.2 Tariffs

developed faster. It works closely with the Health Agency and can propose appropriate measures to the Minister of Health to combat diseases.

4.5.2.1 Tasks in a pandemic

For pandemics, the Institute prepares risk analyses for different pathogens.[35] These analyses should show how long the pandemic will last and when it will cause what damage to which persons and companies. The ministries of labour, economy and digital affairs support the institute in its work by providing data and forecasts.

In a pandemic, the Institute for Diseases and Vaccines ensures cooperation with the Ministry of Security. It determines appropriate protective measures, equipment, tests, medicines and vaccines. The Ministry of Security coordinates production and distribution to the population. It coordinates research and development and provides early support for the licensing procedures for vaccines, medicines and tests in cooperation with the Company Auditing Agency's health auditors. In the case of medicines, it is supported by the Institute of Drugs and Food.

The Institute for Diseases and Vaccines provides the Minister of Health and the population with the collected data on the current infection situation. Testing laboratories, vaccination centres, doctors' surgeries, pharmacies, hospitals and sewage treatment plants report all their data on the pandemic directly to it via the Health Directory. The current situation of the regional infection incidence is measured via the wastewater from households in the sewage treatment plants.

Depending on the infection situation, the Institute determines 3 levels of isolation and infection control measures. At the first level, only protective measures on persons and in companies are prescribed. At the second level, certain companies are closed and activities banned. At the third level, curfews, travel bans and home work are imposed and all public institutions are closed. The measures of each level are to be continuously adjusted during the pandemic only if the other measures

---

35http://dipbt.bundestag.de/dip21/btd/17/120/1712051.pdf

have become too ineffective. The population should not be continually re-acclimatised in order to be able to re-establish a daily routine and habits as quickly as possible.

A vaccine is a medicine that makes the human to whom it is administered immune to the disease and prevents him from passing it on. In other words, it must not make him sick or be infectious. After a test phase of at least 12 months with at least 500,000 test patients, the vaccine may be released. Of the test patients, a maximum of 500 test patients may experience severe side effects. Both the test patients and all those vaccinated are asked to report their health status monthly via the Health Directory. If severe or long-lasting side effects occur with a frequency of more than 0.1%, the vaccine will be banned. The same procedure applies to medicines. Anyone who wishes to report voluntarily as a test patient can do so through the Health Directory. The same procedure that applies to vaccines also applies to medicines against the pandemic disease.

The compulsory or necessary administration of vaccines or medicines is not permitted. Humans have the right to fall ill and die. They make a note on their Health Card with any physician that they do not wish to be vaccinated or treated. In doing so, they can give specific information about one or more particular vaccines, medicines or treatments. In the event of hospital overcrowding, those patients who have opted out of vaccination, medication or treatment will first be denied treatment for the pandemic disease. In a further sorting out of patients by physicians, the So-called triaging, patients with poorer chances of survival and higher age will be turned away first.

At the beginning of the pandemic, the scientific scenarios created on the course of a pandemic are published and filmed so that the population knows what to expect and for how long. For this purpose, the Institute works together with Government Television[36] and Party Television .[37]

---

36 Ministry of Media - 7 Government Television
37 Ministry of Media - 10 Party Television

4.5.3 Institute for Toxic and Hazardous Substances

The Institute for Toxic and Hazardous Substances investigates which substances are toxic or harmful to humans. It examines the samples it receives from Company Auditing Agency auditors, physicians or patients. The Institute tests suspected harmful products and substances and researches agents that can neutralise poisons and hazardous substances or replace them in a way that is safe for health.

It forwards the information to the Health Agency, which formulates it into requirements for the companies and introduces it as a bill in voting with the Minister of Health. The health auditors monitor compliance with the requirements.

4.5.4 Institute for Environmental Health

The Ministry of Health maintains the Institute of Environmental Health, which tests all substances for their environmental compatibility, labels environmentally hazardous goods and proposes regularisations for the handling of these substances. The health auditors collect the necessary samples, physicians and agronomists of the Institute evaluate the samples. Data from the technical auditors from their inspections of work equipment, goods and services are also included in the evaluation.

For substances that are harmful to humans and nature in the long run, alternatives are researched that are not harmful, or recycling techniques that make harmful substances disposable. These proposals are sent to the companies and rated by entrepreneurs and employees and improved if necessary. Domestic entrepreneurs who produce the affected substances receive the results free of charge, but must adapt their performance accordingly. If necessary, the Institute can recommend to the Minister of Health to ban the harmful work equipment, goods and services by law.

The researchers are investigating how long raw materials need to grow back and how long artificial substances need to be degraded until they are environmentally sustainable.

The institute is researching new ways to process pollutants

in such a way that they become environmentally friendly or can be recycled as raw materials. Its goal is to make an environmentally neutral economy possible. Environmentally neutral means existing in such a way that after disappearing, nature is no more polluted than before. All business processes that burden nature must be avoided or processed for disposal and recycling, up to and including environmentally compatible substances. Environmentally compatible substances can be degraded by nature in the open air within 100 years.

The institute researches how the import of pathogens, non-native animals and plants may possibly, currently or in the future affect the local ecosystem. It makes recommendations to Customs[38] on which imports of which organisms, goods or persons should be restricted, banned or controlled for pests and diseases and how precisely. In the event of a possible threat to the local ecosystem, a full inspection of all goods and persons may be recommended instead of random sampling.

4.5.5 Institute for Occupational Health

The University Hospital in the capital city of the Ministry of Health maintains an institute for occupational health that researches the effects of working conditions on the human body and explores new alternatives for harmful working conditions that are not harmful or can significantly reduce the damage. This work involves physicians, hospitals, university clinics, companies and workers. The Institute for Evaluation of Occupational Health analyses the data from the health auditors and combines it with data on occupational accidents or diseases to identify companies, industries and working conditions that pose a risk to workers.

Companies, industries and employees who fall into the risk group are asked by the health auditors to make proposals in questionnaires, which are forwarded to the Institute of Occupational Health. Together with engineers from Planned Economy, Social Market Economy[39] , the ministries of education and innovation and the technical auditors of the

38 Ministry of Security - 8 Customs
39 Ministry of Social Market Economy

Company Auditing Agency, new working tools are developed that improve working conditions. These proposals are sent to suitable companies, rated by entrepreneurs and employees and improved if necessary. Domestic companies that produce work tools receive the results free of charge, but must adapt their work tools to them.

Permanently harmful work for the human body that cannot be changed or automated is being sought together with the Institute for Education[40] so that workers can change professions after a certain age. The Institute for Occupational Health is looking for occupations that are gentle and stressful so that companies can find suitable partners for takeover agreements.[41] Workers and entrepreneurs report to the health auditors if the occupation can no longer be practised after a certain age. Health examinations are then carried out on voluntary workers in the affected occupations and the strain is assessed by doctors.

5 Health care

The Ministry of Health provides health care for the population through physicians, physician assistants, nurses and pharmacists in health and care facilities. The pharmaceutical industry provides the necessary equipment for health care and the production of drugs for the population. Health care is financed by health insurance funds and a uniform medical fee schedule. The Ministry of Health uses the Health Agency and the health auditors of the Company Auditing Agency to check compliance with all requirements.

The principle is: "He who heals is right" and "There is no right to life at any price". In the short term, no life-sustaining measures will be performed after the age of 80, in the medium term after the age of 100, and in the long term after the age of 120, unless one is insured under the Immortality Health Insurance. The age limits are set by the people in a committee.

---

40 Ministry of Education - 4.7 Institute of Education
41 Ministry of Labour - 12.2.6 Transfer agreement for older employees

5.1 Visit to the physician

Patients can visit physicians to have their health condition diagnosed and undergo appropriate treatment. Patients are free to choose the physician they wish to be treated by. To see a physician, patients need an appointment unless it is an emergency.

An emergency is characterised by imminent danger. This is the case when delaying treatment will permanently worsen the state of health. In an emergency, patients can go to the emergency room of a hospital or to a doctor's office without an appointment. Provided patients come without an appointment and are not an emergency, the physician has the right to ask these patients for an appointment and send them away again.

Patients can get an appointment in person, by phone or via the Health Directory. In the Health Directory, they can enter their symptoms so that suitable physicians are automatically displayed. In addition, they can also select physicians who are suitable for them.

5.1.1 Selection of the treatment method

Each patient is entitled to up to 3 opinions from different physicians. If patients intend to get more than one opinion, they must indicate this when they visit the doctor. To get an opinion, a physician makes a diagnosis and proposes his or her treatment method. Patients can then check whether the diagnoses are the same everywhere and which treatment method they would prefer to undergo. The Health Directory helps them make this decision. They can check for which symptoms and diagnoses the treatment method is used and how successfully the selected physician uses this treatment method.

The patient must decide on a treatment method with one physician. Simultaneous treatment by more than one physician is prohibited. For verification purposes, physicians are notified when the Health Card is scanned if a patient is already being treated by another physician for the same symptoms. They have the duty to refuse treatment unless the patient pays for the treatment himself. Only when a treatment method has been completed and the patient's symptoms persist in whole or in part, may another physician treat with a different treatment method.

5.1.2 Responsibility

Which physicians are responsible is shown to the patient when searching the Health Directory. Physicians must be approved by the health auditors in order to be allowed to treat certain symptoms. The Medical Fee Schedule regulates which symptoms these are. There, symptoms are connected with diagnoses, treatment methods and prices. After a diagnosis, physicians can issue prescriptions for treatment, with which the patient can obtain the necessary medicines from a pharmacy or receive them directly from the physician. The physician can then use the prescription to reorder the appropriate amount of medicine. If the physician is not able to export all or part of the treatment, he or she can issue a referral to another physician, whom the patient should then visit. A certain number of appointments may be noted on the referral for doctor visits based on referrals.

5.2 Health Card[42]

Every citizen receives a standardised health insurance card from his or her health insurance fund, the So-called Health Card. The card is the size of an electronic cash card and has a magnetic strip and an internal memory that can be accessed with a card reader. The functions of the Health Card can also be expelled on the identity card. Each citizen decides for himself whether he wants a Health Card or whether he wants to bundle all functions in his identity card. Access to a person's complete non-anonymised data is only available to the attending physician, the affected patient and, in the case of litigation and prevention of danger, also to the Ministry

---

42§236,6,7 Health care: KV Art.41, §241,4 Transplantation medicine

of Health. Any commercial access and use is prohibited. Violations are punishable by at least 5 years' detention. Only the patient is entitled to publish his or her data in the Health Directory in order to participate in the improvement and research of treatments and medicines.

The Health Card stores the name, address, date of birth, weight, eye colour, hair colour, vaccination certificate, X-ray certificate, organ and blood donor card, blood group and living will. In addition, the link to the storage location in the People's Computer[43] are also stored there for the findings, diagnoses, pictures, reports, prescriptions of all previous illnesses and the referrals to other physicians. All physicians who treat a patient can access the data in the People's Computer via the Intranet and automatically leave an entry in the access log of the Access Directory[44] .

Through the patient's history, the physician has a better picture with comprehensive material about the weak points and strengths of that patient's body. This reduces consultation time and makes virtual doctor visits easier. In addition, a patient who is unresponsive in an emergency can be treated more appropriately and quickly, or in the case of death, blood or organs can be collected more quickly. Physicians and pharmacists can use the map to see which medicines are still being taken and to detect and avoid interactions.

Every Health Card holder can access the living will and organ donation details via their People's Computer. Organ donation of all organs and blood donation after death are permitted as default settings. Also stored is a living will that excludes life-sustaining measures for more than 7 days. The holder can edit the information at any time.

5.3 Health Directory[45]

The Ministry of Health operates the Health Directory to unite the diverse tasks for patients, physicians, pharmacists and researchers on a digital platform. For the physician, the

---

43 Ministry of Digital Affairs - 13.6 People's Computers
44 Ministry of Digital Affairs - 7.5 Access Directory
45 §236,6,8 Public health: KV Art.41, §238,2 Alternative medicine

Health Directory is an appointment calendar, index card and billing programme all in one. For health insurers, it is the administration programme for their clients. For the pharmaceutical industry, it is the test programme for their products.

In the Health Directory, all institutions that support the health of persons have a profile. The profile indicates whether the facility is a freelance physician without an office, a medical practice, a hospital or a pharmacy. Each person working in the health sector must be assigned to at least one profile. The necessary data is imported from the person's profile in the Labour Directory. The groups are the respective specialties, subgroups are individual fields of activity within a specialty. For example, orthopaedics would be a group and physiotherapy a subgroup. Record entries can be recorded by the attending staff via camera and microphone and automatically transcribed. The staff then confirms or corrects the automatic entries. In case of doubt, the education and the spoken word are valid.

All persons providing treatment settle their costs with the health insurance companies via the Health Directory. No other form of billing is permitted, as the Company Auditing Agency uses this data for its audits. In the case of cash payment and the express wish of a patient, an entry in the Health Directory can be waived.

New alternative medicine or advanced treatment pathways must apply to the Company Auditing Agency's health auditors and pay for this audit in order to be included in the Health Directory.

5.3.1 Selection

Searches can be made by name, specialty and postcode district. Patients can make an appointment via the Health Directory, thanks to synchronised calendar function. The calendar function is the interface for scheduling appointments, templates for patient records and treatment measures, and a digital archive. The calendar function also makes it possible to look into the past of this health facility. A sorting function makes it possible to search and sort the data of the calendar functions of all health care facilities in order to give patients, physicians, pharmacists and researchers an overview of the effectiveness in combating a disease.

The Health Directory serves consumer policy in the health sector. Patients can search for physicians, practices, hospitals and pharmacies and enter experiences with and ratings about doctors, pharmacists, medicines and treatments.

5.3.2 Quality control

Physicians must create a digital file for each patient. In it, they enter their diagnoses, treatments and prescribed medicines. Pharmacists enter all medicines and drugs sold to these patients. Physicians must mark patients as recovered when they have successfully completed treatment. Patients can also mark themselves as recovered if they feel well after treatment. This indication of patients can be done before or after the physician marks them as recovered.

Patients should report side effects of treatments and medicines. If they report them to the physician or pharmacist, he or she reviews them and is obliged to make an entry in the Health Directory. Voluntary entries by patients are good and bad experiences with treatment persons and methods, medicines, side effects and interactions. Each medicine and each person treating it can be given a rating of up to six stars, which mean anything from "heals quickly" to "does not heal at all". The Health Agency checks entries from patients who have not previously been checked by a physician.

5.3.3 Data release

It is up to each patient to decide how much personal data to publish in the Health Directory. The patient data is displayed anonymously in public. In the public display, the name, address and any contact details are anonymised. Gender, year and month of birth, height, weight, blood group, previous illnesses, diagnoses, treatments, medications, operations and the period from illness to recovery in days as well as the total price are displayed.

Patients themselves can view all data collected about them personally and share it with attending physicians or pharmacists by allowing it to be linked to their Health Card. The Company Auditing Agency's health auditors can view all data. For each data retrieval by a treating person or a state employee, an entry is made in the Access Directory.

5.3.4 Example view

Personal data *voluntary*	Symptoms	Diagnosis	Treatment	Medication	Total price	Recovery period
- Bicycle accident on 15.03.2000 - *Mr. Mustermann* - 54 years - 178 cm - 78 kg - Blood group A rh+ - Organ donors except kidneys - Type A diabetic - Long-term medication: OMNICAN Insulinspr.1 ml by Braun - Herniated disc in the 3rd thoracic vertebra	Severe pain in the right leg, immobility of the leg, bleeding wound, below the knee the leg sticks out to the right side	Open splinter fracture of the lower leg of the calf	X-ray, Operation, Plaster, Physiotherapy	Ibuprophen 600 from Stada 25 tablets (painkillers) One tablet per day until the pack is empty.	836 Dollars	16.03. 2000 until 27.06. 2000

5.3.5 Personal data

The personal data is imported from the Health Card and from past visits to the physician or pharmacist. The patient can choose which additional data to provide and whether to leave a comment about symptoms, diagnosis, treatment, medication, price or recovery period.

5.3.6 Symptoms

Symptoms are all the complaints a patient tells the physician while describing their condition. While the physician enters the symptoms, an algorithm searches the database for diagnoses made by other physicians when similar patients described similar symptoms to them. This is the Health Directory's probability calculator. Its results are also displayed to the patient. However, it is up to the physician to decide which diagnosis he or she actually makes. If there is a strong discrepancy, the physician must justify in the findings why he or she made this diagnosis and not another.
To facilitate the physician's writing work, diagnosis suggestions can be accepted directly and the prefabricated texts then only have to be adapted to the patient, if this is still necessary. The physician is shown which treatments and medications were most frequently used by other physicians and most frequently led to the fastest recovery in similar diseases. The physician can use the patient's identity as a filter, in which all the patient's personal data on the intranet are used. The algorithm now only accesses data from similar patients. As a result, only similar persons, for example in weight, appeal, age or gender, are displayed. Possible side effects or interactions are automatically displayed in a warning.

5.3.7 Diagnosis

In the case of diseases, a diagnosis follows; in the case of a routine examination in which nothing is found, the diagnosis is "without findings" or a disease can be ruled out. For each diagnosis, an explanation is filed, which is kept up to date by the Ministry of Education and its university hospitals and is written in a way that is understandable for lay people. Possible symptoms are also indexed there so that one can see how many other diagnoses the symptom would fit. The basis for this database of diagnoses in the Health Directory and their coding is the International Statistical Classification of Diseases and Related Health Problems (ICD)[46] .

5.3.8 Treatment

Treatments are displayed as a keyword. The keyword is provided with a link that can be used to access the matching video in the Knowledge Directory. These videos are produced by the Ministry of Media Affairs[47] . If the treatment does not proceed as in a textbook, the person treating the patient must have his or her treatment checked by the health auditors, and in doing so can produce a video that is sent by the health auditors to medical television. It is crucial that patients can see in advance what they are in for, what will be done to them, under anaesthesia if necessary, what devices will be used and what the premises will look like. Patients can rate and comment on any treatment they have personally enjoyed with up to 6 stars.

5.3.9 Medication

All medicines prescribed to the patient are listed and how often which dosage should be administered. If necessary, instructions for interactions must be followed for the patient personally. The physician or pharmacist informs the patient whether special instructions are to be followed, because an

---

46 https://www.who.int/standards/classifications/classification-of-diseases
47 Ministry of Media Affairs - 10.1.1.5 Medical Television

automatic data comparison is made with the Health Card and all entries of this patient in the Health Directory. For example, a medicine may have the wrong effect if other medicines or drugs are taken regularly but the patient does not want to inform the physician or pharmacist out of ignorance or shame. Therefore, physicians and pharmacists are obliged to maintain secrecy and discretion. The patient can give a rating of up to six stars and a comment for each medicine individually.

5.3.10 Total price

The total price is calculated from all billing figures according to the Medical Fee Schedule and the prices for the medicines as well as privately paid pre-main and follow-up examinations. With personal access, you are shown what percentage of the invoice amount you have to pay yourself and how far away you are until you have to pay the next level of the annual deductible.

5.3.11 Recovery period

The recovery period indicates when the patient falls ill and when he or she recovers. The time of illness is recorded by the physician or the person treating the patient. The recovery period is recorded by the patient and automatically requested by the Health Directory so that it is not forgotten. If one does not want to use a People's Computer, one must call the physician or the person treating the patient to make the entry. If the treatment is completed with a newly appointment, where the recovery is checked by a physician, the physician must confirm the recovery.

5.3.12 Gene database

Death is the last entry a physician makes about a patient in the Health Directory. As soon as a physician establishes death and issues the digital death certificate, a gene sample is taken. For this purpose, a few hairs with hair roots are pulled out and sent to the gene pool in the Ministry of Health together with the personal data. There, the genetic material is sequenced and created as a file. The genetic samples are barcoded and archived in a refrigerated place. This repository of the domestic gene pool is located in the capital city of the Ministry of Health. The file in the gene database contains all the data from the intranet directories on the person and the genetic code. If, over time, genetic traits become extinct or resistance to disease is sought, an algorithm can automatically search all the genetic information of all the deceased, display matching genetic samples and their storage location.

5.4 Physicians

A physician is any person who has received a licence from the health auditors to treat patients. In principle, a distinction is made between doctors and healers, but transitions are possible. While professional training for doctors is prescribed by the state, healers may be qualified according to their own or traditional training courses. Doctors can follow training courses of healers and vice versa. Therefore, all persons who are able to heal humans are considered physicians. Persons who attend to patients and care for them according to the instructions of a physician are considered physician assistants. Physicians make diagnoses to determine or rule out a disease. Physicians treat their patients until they are well, discontinue treatment or until the physicians discontinue treatment due to lack of prospects of success or professional knowledge. The Medical Fee Schedule applies to the remuneration of physicians through the health insurance funds. Physicians are subject to a working time limit of no more than 14 hours per day, followed by a non-working time of at least 10 hours. Physicians may perform their services at patients' homes, remotely via digital means, in physicians' offices or hospitals.

5.4.1 Approval[48]

The professional law for physicians regulates licensing. The Company Auditing Agency's health auditors' examination for licensing as a physician tests the degree or successful method of healing. Physicians receive a profile in the Health Directory with their state-approved degree or after being approved by the health auditors, which they can link to a practice, hospital or university clinic, depending on where they are currently working. They can activate this profile in the Labour Directory to search for jobs or to have potential employers find them.

During their medical career, physicians are audited every 2 years by health auditors. During these audits, professional treatment is checked by undercover investigators and test patients. Undercover investigators are health auditors who are trained physicians or physician assistants and work with the physician being audited. Test patients are patients who are selected and paid by the health auditors to be treated by the physician being audited and newly examined by a physician selected by the health auditors after each visit to the physician. In addition, all continuing education certificates are checked in the regular announced examinations. Physicians are obliged to attend at least one continuing education course in their specialist department every 2 years. If physicians are insufficiently examined 3 times in a row or if there are more than 10 complaints between 2 examinations, the health auditors withdraw the licence of the affected physician. The physician can appeal to the courts. If the court confirms the withdrawal of the licence, a temporary or permanent occupational ban can be imposed.

5.4.1.1 Doctors

A doctor is someone who has successfully completed medical studies. The completed medical studies qualify graduates to practise general medicine. They are entitled to open a practice or a hospital. Following the medical studies, the So-called medical specialist can be made. This further training is part-

---

48§236.5a Health Care: BV Art. 117a

time and is completed with a theoretical and practical final examination. Specialists are specialised in one field of medicine and can set up specialist practices or specialist departments in hospitals or open such institutions.

Those who have a foreign degree must take the final examination of their medical studies at a domestic college and are then allowed to practise. Further study is then no longer necessary. If the final examination is failed more than 2 times, the examinee must complete the medical studies at a domestic college.

5.4.1.2 Medical assistant

You are considered a physician assistant if you directly assist a physician or provide care and assistance to patients yourself. For example, opticians, nurses, outpatient or inpatient care workers are considered physician assistants. These are all those persons who have received the appropriate referral from a physician and who have a recognised training[49] . Training as a physician assistant is an educational programme at state colleges. Physician assistants also have a duty of confidentiality and a duty of disclosure equivalent to that of a physician. There is only a duty to treat if the physician prescribes treatment to fulfil it.

5.4.1.3 Healer[50]

You are considered a healer if you can prove that you have healed at least 100 persons through your treatments. This proof must be provided during the licensing examination by the health auditors of the Company Auditing Agency. Proof is deemed to be provided if the treatment methods, medication if applicable and the recovery period are stated. The treated patients must have been to a physician prior to this, who establishes their illness through an appropriate diagnosis. After treatment with the healer and recovery, the patient

---

49 Ministry of Education - 4.8 Recognition of qualifications
50 §236,3,5a Health care: KV Art.41, BV Art. 117a, §238 Alternative medicine: BV Art. 118a

has to go back to the physician who now has to determine their recovery. This process is necessary for all 100 patients required for examination admission. The 100 patients treated must have been to at least 25 different physicians. The health auditors visit at least three different treatments of the healer, but at least as many until all methods of the healer have been looked at once and documented by video. The health auditors send at least one test patient and professionals from the university hospitals who are trained in the speciality and check the diagnosis and recovery of at least 10 patients. On passing the exam, the healer gets accreditation and a profile in the Health Directory. Until the first 100 patients are accredited and treated, the healer is considered a "probationary healer".

5.4.1.4 Public health officers

Public health officers are all physicians who work in the service of the Health Agency, university hospitals and health auditors. They check the work of other physicians and may be called upon as assessors in court proceedings. Through their regular audits of physicians and patients treated, they replace the medical departments of the state health insurance funds, which are only responsible for the administration of contributions and disbursements. The legality of the treatment costs is guaranteed by the review. This verification uses all patient data from the Health Directory. An algorithm shows auditors similar patients with similar symptoms and diagnoses, what treatment steps and medications followed, how these services could be billed under the Medical Fee Schedule and what fees were actually billed, as well as all comments and ratings from patients since the last audit. If auditors find irregularities, they question the affected physicians as to why other physicians treated similar patients and the same diagnoses differently. In case of doubt, the patient is questioned personally. Patients with complaints about physicians and physician assistants have the opportunity to make comments and ratings in the Health Directory or to contact the Company Auditing Agency directly at any time. Every complaint is addressed at the regular review, which takes place every 2 years. If complaints accumulate with a treating physician or physician assistant, this is noted as a deficiency in the audit report, which must be remedied by the next audit. If the deficiency persists, the licence is withdrawn for 12 months. If the deficiency is serious and irreparable, the licence is withdrawn completely. Legal process is possible.

5.4.1.5 Paediatricians

Paediatricians and children's hospitals treat all children living inland until they reach the age of majority. There are compulsory preventive medical check-ups and vaccinations for children. Children also receive a Health Card from the General Health Insurance with their child ID card, through which paediatricians settle their fees. Health insurance contributions are paid through child benefits. Parents are obliged to have all child check-ups[51] and vaccinations against childhood diseases. Vaccinations are basically voluntary, but as soon as children can speak, they decide whether they want to be vaccinated or not after an educational discussion with the paediatrician.

Paediatricians are also employees of the Youth Welfare Office. They have a duty of confidentiality, but also a duty to report, treat and notify. The duty of confidentiality is the same as for other physicians, but here the parents of the child and employees of the Youth Welfare Office are excluded. The duty to report also corresponds to that of other physicians, but here the parents are taken to court. Paediatricians always have a duty to treat, but they have the right to expel relatives with insubordinate behaviour and to pick up the child outside the practice or hospital after treatment. Paediatricians also have a duty to report to the Youth Welfare Office as soon as they recognise physical abuse and external or mental neglect. In acute cases of child endangerment, paediatricians have the right to inform the police and the Youth Welfare Office in

---

51 https://www.bundesgesundheitsministerium.de/u-untersuchung.html

order to have children taken into state care immediately.[52]

5.4.1.6 Veterinarians and herbalists

Physicians for animals or plants are considered to be physicians who have completed appropriate training and healers who have been successfully audited. Owners of animals and plants have the option of taking out health insurance for their property and can bill medical visits via the Medical Fee Schedule. Physicians for animals and plants, like all physicians, are subject to the duty of disclosure and confidentiality. They are not subject to compulsory treatment. However, they are subject to the duty to report if they recognise that keepers are keeping their animals or plants improperly or torturing them, as well as if animals or plants are afflicted with diseases that may become epidemics. They can admonish the keepers or make a report to the Health Agency. In the case of private individuals, the Health Agency checks the conditions and in the case of companies, the health auditors of the Company Auditing Agency do so. If it is proven that the welfare of animals or plants is being violated, the animals may be confiscated. Animals are then sent to an animal shelter and plants to nurseries or market gardens.

5.4.2 Duties

Physicians have a duty of confidentiality and a duty of disclosure. The duty of confidentiality means that they do not discuss their patients' illnesses except with the patients themselves or other physicians and physician assistants who also treat, attend or care for the patient.

The obligation to report means that cases of fraud must be reported. If a patient wants to obtain services by fraud, the physician informs the patient. If the patient still wants to be treated, this is noted on the Health Card and sent to the Health Agency. The Health Agency forwards the case of fraud to the nearest public health officer, who can summon

---

52Ministry of Planned Economy - 18.1.7 Children's House

the patient for an examination. If the suspicion of fraud is confirmed, the public health officer forwards the results to the patient's health insurance company, which can use them to charge the patient in court.

Only emergency physicians in ambulances or physicians in the emergency room are obliged to treat patients. All other physicians have the right to turn away patients with insubordinate behaviour or lack of health insurance.

All physicians must comply with medical law, which prescribes a certain handling of patients in medical research, reproduction and transplantation.

5.4.2.1 Medical research[53]

All physicians are part of medical research and all patients participate in studies. A distinction is made between the development of new treatment methods and the quality assurance or improvement of existing treatment methods.

Quality assurance and improvement is ensured by entering all treatment data in the Health Directory. This allows existing treatment methods to be further researched even after they have been approved, in order to discover late effects, side effects or interactions in long-term studies. The success of a treatment method may depend on pre-existing conditions, drug use, lifestyle or the genetic make-up of a patient. In the approval procedures, such a wide range of test patients can never be presented, although this is the only way to confirm or disprove a successful cure. For this reason, physicians are obliged to disclose the methods and results of their treatment together with the personal data of the patients in the Health Directory.

5.4.2.1.1 Research into new treatment methods

The development of new treatments is subject to oversight by the Company Auditing Agency's health auditors. Certain conditions apply under which patients may become test

---

53 §239.2 Research on humans: BV Art. 118b

patients.

Firstly, the research project is checked by the health auditors to see whether the burdens and risks for plants, animals and humans are as low as possible, whether the test subjects and test patients are protected in the best possible way and whether the benefits from the research project justify these burdens and risks. In case of doubt, the milder means must be chosen or a committee convened. In the case of medical research, suitable plants and animals should be selected as test objects first, and only then should research be carried out on humans if it has been proven that they are harmless in animals of the same species. For certain treatment methods, such as psychotherapy or sound therapy, the health auditors can exclude experiments on plants or animals.

Secondly, the persons who could become test patients must be informed by a physician about the procedure and the risks. The content of these explanatory talks must be approved by the health auditors before the talks can be held. It is checked whether the procedure and risks are explained sufficiently and in a way that can be understood by laypersons. Each educational interview must be filmed in full with a camera and saved in the Health Directory. After this interview, the persons must decide whether they want to become test patients or not. There must be at least 24 hours between the interview and the decision. After a refusal, no further action may be taken by physicians, researchers or other personnel involved in the research. A refusal must be accepted as binding. If the person agrees to become a test patient, this consent must be in writing and in the form of a video and must be stored in the Health Directory.

Thirdly, an exception applies to research projects that cannot do without persons who are incapable of making their own judgement. Persons incapable of judgement are characterised by the fact that their physical, mental or health condition prevents them from making a conscious judgement about their consent to participate in the research project. If the expected benefit for the participant is high, the risks and burdens may also be high. If, on the other hand, the expected benefit is low, risks must be minimal and burdens must be reversible. For example, a study on a patient who is in a coma would only be permissible if either no damage can be done to him or her or if there is a certified chance of recovery and the patient has not objected to such treatment in his or her living will.

Fourth, the Company Auditing Agency's health auditors monitor ongoing research through their regular audits of researching companies, institutes and other research organisations.

5.4.2.2 Reproduction[54]

Reproductive medicine protects human dignity, the personality and the family of the parents and the child. This protection is guaranteed by the following requirements.

Sexuality education is already provided in educational institutions.[55] Special sexuality education adapted to the individual is provided by paediatricians, gynaecologists and urologists as part of their medical practice. This applies in particular to suitable contraceptives and to risks for women with health impairments that could lead to damage to the mother or child. For the eradication of hereditary diseases or disabilities, the people may prescribe gene therapy by law in a committee.

5.4.2.2.1 Abortion

The termination of a pregnancy is permitted without restriction up to the 3rd month of pregnancy. Up to the 6th month of pregnancy, it is only permissible if a disability of the child has been detected which was not detectable up to the 3rd month. After that, abortion is only permissible if the mother's life is in danger and can only be saved by it. Paediatricians, gynaecologists or urologists are responsible for giving advice

---

54§240.3 Reproductive medicine and genetic engineering in the human sector: BV Art. 119
55Ministry of Education - 8.7.4.5 Sex Education

to expectant parents and informing them about abortion or confidential birth. They can also refer one or both parents to appropriate counselling centres of the Ministry of Family Affairs. The details are regulated similarly to the Pregnancy Conflict Act.[56]

5.4.2.2.2 Inability to conceive

If a parent is unable to reproduce for health reasons, a physician can provide medical assistance for involuntary childlessness. This means using the parents' egg and sperm for artificial insemination, using an egg or sperm donation from the egg and sperm bank, or using a surrogate mother. Women of childbearing age can register with their gynaecologist as a surrogate mother and donate eggs. Surrogacy and egg donation must be voluntary and unpaid. Men can make a sperm donation at their urologist's office. Sperm donation must be voluntary and unpaid. Surrogate mothers, egg donors and sperm donors are listed in a database from which patients can select the most suitable person. As owners of their data, surrogate mothers, egg or sperm donors can hide all or part of their data. The egg and sperm banks are located in university hospitals.

5.4.2.2.3 Genetic test

General practitioners are responsible for carrying out genetic tests on patients who expressly request this and confirm their wish in writing. In these genetic tests, the genetic material is taken, examined, stored and shown to the patient as a result. The examination may cover hereditary diseases, genetic defects and parentage. Anyone who has a genetic test carried out thereby votes in favour of storage in the gene database. The data in this gene pool can be used to trace hereditary diseases and ancestry.

During pregnancy, a genetic test may be carried out up to the 3rd and, if it is not medically possible by then, also up to

56http://www.gesetze-im-internet.de/beratungsg/BJNR113980992.html

the 6th month of pregnancy. The purpose of this genetic test is to determine, with the help of current genetic diagnostics, whether the child suffers from a hereditary disease or a genetic defect that could lead to a disability. The father and mother must agree to the genetic test. If the genetic test reveals a hereditary disease or a genetic defect, the pregnancy may be terminated up to the completion of the 6th month of pregnancy.

5.4.2.2.4 Identity of the parents

Mothers are obliged to declare their identity and that of the father at the time of birth. If they do not know the identity of the father beyond doubt, they must provide the personal data of all possible fathers. The Health Agency is responsible for finding the father and carrying out a paternity test on presumed fathers. If the father does not wish to reveal his identity to the mother, he must inform the Health Agency in writing. In any case, a child has a right to know the identity of its parents. Mothers must register a confidential birth with the Health Agency. They must then give one or more male and female first names and choose a pseudonym for themselves. The pseudonym consists of an invented first and last name of the mother. She can give birth under this name in any hospital or with a physician in a home birth. The child bears the given first name and the surname of the pseudonym. At the latest when the child reaches the age of majority, the Health Agency reveals to him or her who his or her biological parents are. The same applies to egg and sperm donors.

5.4.2.3 Transplantation[57]

Transplantation medicine involves the medical removal of organs, tissues and cells from one body and transplantation into another. It can be applied to plants, animals and humans. In the case of humans, the protection of human dignity, personality and the health of the donor and recipient applies.

57§241,1,2,3 Transplantation medicine: BV Art. 119a

Protection is considered to be guaranteed if the following conditions are met. In the event of a shortage, organs are given priority to recipients who have not yet reached the age of 70, who are in the worst health and who are expected to be in the best health after the transplant. The trade and marketing of organs, tissues and cells in return for payment or a service are prohibited. Exceptions apply to animal or artificially cultured organs, tissues and cells. Artificial cultivation may not take place in any body that has consciousness.

5.4.3 Physicians' association

The physicians' association shall consist of physicians from university hospitals and representations democratically elected by domestic citizens. The physicians' association shall have representatives for each specialist department who are able to assess the workload and the prospects of success of treatments for certain symptoms and diagnoses. The physicians' association shall lobby for the interests of physicians and represent the medical profession in a committee. If its representations participate in legislative processes, even if only for advisory purposes, the rules for lobbyists apply. The medical association has a profile in the Lobby Directory.[58]

5.4.4 Triaging

In a triaging process, those providing assistance must choose the order of priority in which patients are treated. In cases of severe illness or injury and insufficient availability of equipment or personnel, lower-ranking treatment then leads to death or permanent damage. Who may make this decision and when, based on what conditions, is formulated by an ethics committee and a committee and submitted to the people for a vote.[59]

Firstly, those who refuse suitable treatment methods and

---

58 Ministry of State Organisation - 9.10.10 Lobbyists in the legislative process
59 Ministry of State Organisation - 8.5.9 Ethics Commission, 9.10.11.3 Direct legislation

thereby deliberately and knowingly reduce their chances of survival are given lower priority. Such deciders are stored as living wills on the Health Card. Secondly, those who have lower chances of survival are given lower priority. The assessment of the chances of survival is made jointly by three physicians in a hospital and, at the scene of an accident, by the first rescue worker who is able to do so. Thirdly, whoever is older is given lower priority. The deciding factor in triaging is the data on the Health Card. Only in an emergency are rescue workers allowed to do without it.

In the case of accidents, there are usually too few rescue workers on the scene immediately. All patients whose lives are not in danger should seek outpatient or inpatient treatment themselves. Those who cannot do so should wait for transport. Patients whose lives are in danger are marked. The patients who have the best chance of survival are to be supported first. If the chances are considered equal, age is the deciding factor. Rescue workers can read the Health Card via a reader to view living wills and health data. If a living will refuses rescue, the patient will not be treated at all unless he revokes his living will to the rescue forces.

During waves of disease, disasters or pandemics, hospitals and other treatment facilities can become so overloaded that triaging is necessary. In order to prevent such triaging, the Ministry of Health has the duty to transfer the healthcare system into an extraordinary situation for a limited period of time. During the extraordinary situation, the Minister of Health, or in the case of municipal affected, the deputy Minister of Health, has special rights. The special rights enable all appropriate forces from the Ministries of Security, Infrastructure and Planned Economy to be called in to assist.

In the case of treatment outside the Medical Fee Schedule and lack of insurance cover by Immortality Health Insurance, treatment will also be discontinued.

5.5 Medical Fee Schedule[60]

In the Medical Fee Schedule, prices are set for treatments provided by physicians or physician assistants. Its structure is similar in detail to the German Medical Fee Schedule.[61] The aim of the Medical Fee Schedule is to provide medical care for all citizens so that communicable, common and fatal diseases are cured or their courses are made more bearable for patients. Under this fee schedule, physicians can bill health insurance companies for their services. The Medical Fee Schedule applies to humans as well as to keepers of animals and plants. All physicians who are licensed are obliged to offer the services of the Medical Fee Schedule of their specialist department, although not necessarily at the prescribed prices.

The prices may be multiplied by factors and thereby reduced or increased. Factors shall be applied whenever the difficulty of the treatment differs from a method of treatment assumed to be normal due to an increased or decreased expenditure of time, personnel and material. Prices may also be increased by surcharges if treatment takes place outside the regular duty period, outside the regular duty station or without an appointment because it constitutes an emergency.

For example, a physician may make a home visit because the patient cannot go to the doctor's office or hospital. Suppose the home visit is due to an emergency on a public holiday shortly after midnight and the treatment requires a physician's assistant, a special device and medicine. During the treatment, a complication arises because the patient has developed a concomitant disease. Moreover, he does not understand the physician's language well because the national language is not his mother tongue. In this case, the highest factor is applied because the treatment requires more time, staff and material. Surcharges would apply for emergency, home visit, holiday work and night work.

Physicians also have the right to offer additional services outside of the Medical Fee Schedule and to offer services from the Medical Fee Schedule at specially set prices. In these two

60 §236.5b Public health: BV Art. 117a, §237.2b Protection of health and environment: BV Art. 118
61 http://www.gesetze-im-internet.de/go__1982/

cases, the state health insurance funds do not cover the costs of such treatments. The patient must now bear the additional costs himself. Physicians are obliged to inform patients about the cost price before treatment and to treat patients only after they have given their consent. The consent has to be proven by a written treaty and can be checked by the health auditors. Services outside the Medical Fee Schedule or services from the Medical Fee Schedule with other prices must also be documented in the Health Directory. The health auditors monitor the frequency of use of non-Medical Fee Schedule services and propose their inclusion in the Medical Fee Schedule to the Minister of Health. They also monitor independent pricing by physicians and use by patients and propose a price adjustment to the Minister of Health.

5.5.1 Price negotiations

The Medical Fee Schedule is a law that affects physicians because it interferes with their free pricing and thus with economic freedom. As soon as the affected citizens trigger the repeal quorum[62] , the law is newly negotiated. These price negotiations are held as a committee and concluded by voting. Those entitled to vote are all physicians. On the panel are representatives of the health insurance companies, the medical association, the Health Agency, the health auditor and the Minister of Health. The audience includes physicians from all specialties who have been elected as experts by the members of the Medical Association. The committee is broadcast in real time on Government Television[63] so that all physicians can participate in the negotiation through their People's Computers. In the price negotiations, all treatment methods are presented one by one and a price is set. For each diagnosis and its treatments, the appropriate professionals come to the panel and describe what actions, devices and medicines are needed to perform a treatment. Then the time, materials and training required are calculated. Proposed prices are adopted, decided with the agreement of all panelists and a majority vote

---

62 Ministry of State Organisation - 9.5.15 Repeal quorum
63 Ministry of Media - 7 Government Television

of the audience and viewers. In case of doubt, the Minister of Health has the final decision-making right or can also let the people make this right for one or more decisions.

A special feature in this committee is that the people must approve the law in the budget vote[64] . This exception is justified by the fact that the Medical Fee Schedule concerns health insurance companies and patients and, as a social policy measure, sets the price of health services instead of allowing it to fluctuate freely. When voting by the people, those entitled to vote can adjust individual prices to their liking or reject the overall result. If there is a majority of price adjustments or rejections, the Medical Fee Schedule is newly negotiated in a People's Committee. In these price negotiations, compromises can be reached or exclusions can be made. Compromises mean a price change to the disadvantage of both parties, namely the physicians and the health insurers. The physicians waive a higher price, the health insurers waive a lower price and both parties meet in the middle. If physicians are not willing to lower their prices, health insurers can exclude these treatment methods from insurance coverage. If the people do not agree, health insurance premiums must be increased.

The regular price adjustment automatically uses the inflation rate of the national currency. In this case, there is no need to newly hold a committee. However, if treatment methods change due to technical or scientific progress, a committee must be held. The prices are adjusted to the current conditions. Facilitated treatment methods are reduced in price, new treatment methods are included and priced, obsolete treatment methods are dropped.

5.6 Health facilities[65]

Health care facilities are medical practices, hospitals, state university hospitals and health centres. Physicians can work in practices or hospitals that they operate themselves as entrepreneurs or work there as employees. The Health Agency issues licences for the operation of doctors' practices and

---

64 Ministry of Finance - 9.5 Budget vote
65 §236,2,9,10 Health care: KV Art.41, BV Art. 117a

hospitals and thus ensures sufficient basic medical supply. Licences are therefore not granted if the need is already met. The Health Agency determines the level of need based on the number and demographic structure of the population in the area. The Company Auditing Agency's health auditors check compliance with the standards and thus ensure a consistently high quality of health care. All hospitals are obliged to provide emergency medical care and to be available as the nearest reception point for rescue services.

Physicians may decide to open a practice or hospital in the Social Market Economy or Social Market Economy. In the Social Market Economy, they are subject to the Non-profit principle. Profits must be invested in the quality of treatment or reduced through price discounts. The Health Agency can oblige hospitals to be Non-profit if there are only for-profit hospitals in the region. The treatment catalogue corresponds at least to the services of the Medical Fee Schedule and the prices for these treatments are based exclusively on the Medical Fee Schedule. All patients must be insured in a health insurance scheme that covers the services. Entrepreneurs of the Social Market Economy and their employees are compulsorily insured in the General Health Insurance. Private payments for additional services are allowed and must be made in advance. Those who cannot pay for treatment are allowed to take out a loan from the People's Bank .[66]

No such requirements apply in the Free Market Economy. In particular, the Medical Fee Schedule can be applied there in a limited way or not at all. Physicians are completely free in their pricing and are only bound by contractual requirements that they agree with health insurers or patients. Patients may be insured in a health insurance scheme or have to pay for the treatments privately.

The state hospital system is characterised by health centres[67] and university hospitals. Health centres are operated in Social Villages and capital cities of a Barter Economy Zone[68] . The physicians are employed for an indefinite period of time and

---

66Ministry of Finance - 11 People's Bank
67Ministry of Planned Economy - 18.1.3 Health Centre
68Ministry of Barter Economy - 6 Barter Economy Zone

offer their services under the conditions of the Medical Fee Schedule. There are no additional services there. The patients are residents of the Planned Economy or Barter Economy who manage their health care through taxes. The hospitals in the capital city of a Barter Economy Zone and in the Social Villages of the Planned Economy are also teaching hospitals of the local state college. Thus, the ministries of health and education share the costs.

5.6.1 University hospitals

University hospitals are part of every university and form the subject area of medicine there. In order to be able to train physicians and conduct research, university hospitals offer patients the opportunity to be treated there. The special thing about university hospitals is that they have all the treatment methods available in the domestic healthcare system. Thus, each university hospital consists of medical practices and a hospital with specialists, doctors and healers. Individual university hospitals specialise so that all of them in the alliance can train, offer and research all possibilities of medical treatment.

University hospitals thus fulfil the purpose of being able to relate traditional medicine, alternative medicine and conventional medicine to each other, to identify and test interactions and to develop new combinations of different treatment methods. Patients who receive treatment in university hospitals therefore agree in principle to be used as practice objects for physicians in training and research objects for doctoral students, professors and research assistants. This does not apply to emergency patients who are brought in by the rescue service because the university hospital is the nearest health facility. Known treatments are charged according to the Medical Fee Schedule. New treatments that are being tested are offered at cost price or free of charge.

Physicians at university hospitals alternate between teaching, research and treatment at the university hospital and as health auditors at the Company Auditing Agency. This is to equip physicians at university hospitals with diverse experiences that strengthen their judgement of medical issues. When the state needs to call on experts, such as for committees or judicial assessments, physicians from the appropriate subject areas of a university hospital are called upon. If there are controversial positions, representations from several different university hospitals representing opposing positions are invited. Experts should always be the best in their field. In the selection of the best, the following criteria are taken into account: apt diagnoses and successful treatments, mistreatments, misdiagnoses, research results and the number of times one's own research work has been applied in the professional world.

5.7 Care[69]

Care is intended for humans with disabilities and old age. It is a sub-area of health care that is not designed to make humans healthy again, but to make their complaints more bearable and to enable them to live a life that would not be possible without outside help. The qualifications of care workers are therefore not as demanding as those of physicians and physician assistants. Physicians and physician assistants are only used in care when their expertise is needed. Care workers receive medicine and care instructions from physicians, which are then carried out independently.

Care can be provided by relatives, honorary or professional care workers at the home of the person in need of care or in a nursing home. For outpatient or inpatient care by professional care workers, care insurance must be taken out or the stay must be paid for by the person in need of care themselves. A subsidy from tax funds is excluded. In principle, there is no obligation to take out long-term care insurance. Those in need of care can decide for themselves whether they want to lead such a life or prefer to go to the suicide ward[70] . This decision can also be deposited in a living will on the Health Card if, for example, dementia makes an independent decision impossible.

The Company Auditing Agency's health auditors check that

---

69 §236,3 Health Care: KV Art.41
70 Ministry of Family Affairs - 11.2 Suicide

all companies in the care sector comply with the applicable requirements and serve as a complaints body for those in need of care. The Health Agency issues licences for the operation of outpatient care services and inpatient care homes. It offers advanced training courses for honorary or family caregivers. These courses are led by nurses and physicians who are in training at a state college. They take place outside of school hours in state educational institutions that are located as close as possible to the homes of the participating honorary service or family caregivers. In addition, individual courses can also be attended at the colleges without having to take the course of study.

5.7.1 Care models in the economic forms

Depending on the economic form, there are different care models. In the Barter Economy[71], care services are remunerated with consideration. People in need of care are cared for at home by relatives and friends. Only natural medicines are available, such as medicinal herbal juices or baths, which are common in the Barter Economy. Those who wish to receive modern medical care in the Free Market Economy can take out long-term care insurance while living in the Barter Economy. The prerequisite is that one has saved enough money to be able to pay the premiums.

In Planned Economy, care services are part of the basic supply. People in need of care live in the house for disabled people or in the house for senior citizens and are cared for there by Social Villagers and younger senior citizens. If they become so severely in need of care that they would have to go to a nursing home, they are transferred to the Social Village health centre. The medicines are generic and medicinal herbs from the village's own cultivation. They are provided by a pharmacist, dosed appropriately for a person in need of care by a physician and administered by a physician's assistant who goes from the health centre to the house for disabled people and the retirement home once a day.

In the Social Market Economy, care services are paid for by

71 Ministry of Barter Economy

the long-term care insurance. In the Social Market Economy there is only one long-term care insurance scheme, which is also Non-profit. The contribution is 2.5% of the income of all insured persons and is assessed according to the utilisation of payers and beneficiaries. A deductible is payable, which is based on the need for long-term care. The longer the need for care lasts, the lower the deductible to be paid annually. The difference in the benefits is that family members also receive their care benefits as a fixed monthly amount. This fixed amount depends on the degree of need for care. Persons in need of care are either accommodated at home or in Residential Communities of four persons or more. The Residential Community is preferably housed in a building owned by a person in need of care. Other care recipients pay a rent with which they pay professional care workers and support honorary care workers who can also live in the building, but then do not pay rent. Honorary caregivers are voluntary retirees and roommates. Professional care workers come to each Residential Community once a day by vehicle. Depending on the severity of the disability, people in need of care have to move to care homes, which are organised like the Residential Communities, but are permanently staffed with professional care workers. Nursing robots can also be used as aids in Residential Communities, which make a virtual doctor's consultation possible via video conference or measure bodily functions such as blood pressure, pulse or blood sugar level. The care robots also serve as mobile medicine cabinets that provide the person in need of care with medicine for the day or at the right time or occasion.

In the Free Market Economy, care services are reimbursed by the long-term care insurance companies. The contribution is contractually agreed. People in need of care are cared for on an outpatient basis at home or as inpatients in a nursing home. The individual benefits depend on the treaty between the insured person and the insurance company.

5.7.2 Care levels

The care levels are based on the need for care and differ in terms of caregivers and accommodation. Persons in need of care are those who have a congenital disability, who have become dependent on care due to an accident or illness, or who suffer from age-related illnesses or infirmity. All these different types of impairment can vary in severity, which requires different professional qualifications, regular care visits as well as appropriate accommodation. Where the nature of the impairment allows, care robots are used to approve care workers.

The first stage is care by relatives and friends. They visit the person in need of care weekly or on call in their own home and can participate in further training via the Health Agency. There they learn how to handle the person in need of care and how to remove everyday barriers. People in need of care in the first level can live largely independently. This means at least being able to go to the toilet, wash, dress or get and prepare food themselves. On the other hand, moving loads, putting on certain clothes or the type and speed of locomotion as well as the possibility of movement is restricted.

The second stage is outpatient care by honorary and professional care workers. Honorary service care workers make additional visits to people in need of care at home to approve relatives and friends or to replace absent ones. Professional care workers are there for medical and specialist activities by appointment and on call, which the other voluntary care workers cannot perform. Care recipients in the second stage cannot live independently because at least one daily activity described above cannot be performed. This makes daily visits by a care worker necessary.

The third stage is outpatient care in the family or in a supervised Residential Community. Those in need of care can no longer live alone because they can no longer executive several daily activities. Those who do not have a family who can take them in and care for them at home, rent or buy into Residential Communities. At least 4 persons live together in these communities. About half of the residents should always be in need of care. The others use the discounted living space and, in return, care for and maintain those in need of care, who pay a higher share of the rent. Pets and care robots are also part of the equipment. A professional care worker comes by once a week to take over tasks that no one else in the Residential Community can do.

The fourth stage is inpatient care in a nursing home. Those in need of care can only live so dependent that they have to be cared for around the clock. Honorary and professional care workers are supported by relatives. Nursing homes are a mixture of hospitals and youth hostels. Here, volunteers are only temporarily on duty and professionals are present all the time. In nursing homes, voluntary pensioners or volunteers and pets take care of the daily emotional care of those in need of care. Specialists provide medical, sanitary and technical support to those in need of care. Physicians visit nursing homes weekly and perform the medical treatments that the professionals are unable to perform.

The fifth stage is inpatient care in a hospice. Those who will die within the next 6 months can move into a hospice. Here, the professionals ensure a painless life, but refrain from life-prolonging measures. Lawyers, notaries and undertakers are professionals who visit once a week to prepare the passing. Voluntary helpers, care robots and pets provide emotional care until death.

5.7.3 Care Directory

The Care Directory is used to record the supply and demand for care workers and to distribute them according to need. The number of Residential Communities, Families, Relatives or Honorary Care Workers determines how many professional care workers should be trained and how many care homes should be established or closed.

Each caregiver is given a profile. If they are a professional care worker, their data is imported from their profile in the Labour Directory. Relatives and honorary caregivers create their profile voluntarily and can import further data from other directories. A group is opened for each person in need of care, which is closed again after the person's death. Care facilities such as Residential Communities, Nursing Homes and Hospices form subgroups. The information about the persons in need of care is imported from their profiles in the directories for persons and health and is available in the description of the group. In addition to the necessary information determined by the attending physician, persons in need of care can import further information from their profiles in other directories or enter it themselves. The information shows the care level and what care is necessary for a person in need. The Care Directory automatically links care services, Residential Communities, nursing homes, animal shelters and care robots to the appropriate profiles and groups.

Using a search function, caregivers can select people in need of care and vice versa. Tasks can be distributed via a digital duty roster.[72] Agreements are possible via posts, comments and replies. Caregivers and people in need also have the opportunity to rate each other. Thus, people in need of care can indicate how good they found the treatment and comment on what they particularly noticed. Caregivers, on the other hand, can rate how difficult it is to care for the person in need of care and comment on whether the person is pleasant or defiant.

Another function is the search for Residential Communities and Care Homes. A search function is used to find people in need of care and voluntary carers with similar interests. Persons with similar interests are placed in an institution. In addition, people in need of care can specifically search for other people in need of care who have impairments that balance each other out. This should make it possible to live together with mutual support and little outside help. For example, someone with dementia can still do physical work, while someone with paraplegia can still think perfectly.

5.8 Pharmacist

A pharmacist is anyone who holds a recognised degree in pharmacy. Pharmacists are responsible for the sale of all medicines and drugs and provide advice to purchasers where

---

72Ministry of Planned Economy - 7.6.1 Digital duty roster

a physician has not already done so. Pharmacists can open and run pharmacies. They supply physicians with medicines for direct dispensing to patients. In the case of animals and plants, they sell medicines to the keepers. Pharmacists are particularly able to provide custom-fit medicines and dosages or methods of use for each customer personally.

Medicines that are necessary for medical treatment are covered by the health insurance and paid for with the Health Card. Medicines that do more damage than good when used improperly are subject to prescription. The physician grants the patient purchase authorisations for certain quantities of a medicine via the patient's Health Card and must inform the patient about the exact conditions for taking the medicine. Pharmacists must make sure that the patient is aware of the conditions of use at the time of purchase.

Pharmacists receive information on the consumption of medicines and drugs via the Health Card and warn the patient of side effects, interactions or addiction risks. All medicines sold by pharmacists are stored on the Health Card and in the pharmacy's profile in the Health Directory. This also applies to non-prescription medicines and drugs.

5.8.1 Pharmacists' Association

Pharmacists are organised in an association that purchases medicines, medicines and drugs from the pharmaceutical industry. These collective orders are intended to reduce the price and ensure the availability of all medicines. It represents the interests of pharmacists vis-à-vis the Medical Association, the Pharmaceutical Industry Association and the Ministry of Health. The Pharmacists' Association is responsible for forwarding information on new requirements by the Ministry of Health to pharmacists.

5.9 Medicine[73]

Medicinal products are all medical devices, such as medicines, vaccines or antibiotics, as well as narcotics, such as drugs or painkillers. The Ministry of Health issues the following rules for handling medicines and monitors compliance with them with the help of the health authorities and health auditors of the Company Auditing Agency. In the case of medicines, priority is given to the benefit of humans over animals and plants. Medicines to which pathogens can develop resistance are reserved for humans. All medicines are subject to the purity law, which ensures the highest possible purity from production to trade to consumption. In order to be sold, medicines must be approved by health auditors. In the approval process, the degree of effectiveness and the plant or animal basis are weighed against chemical production. Biodegradable products are preferable to chemical non-degradable or poorly degradable products for the same efficacy. Medicines that cause addiction or damage will have their marketing authorisation withdrawn as soon as research has been carried out into medicines that do not have such side-effects with the same efficacy. The medicines of alternative medicine receive equal attention in studies and approval procedures as those of conventional medicine.

The health auditors, in cooperation with the university hospitals, physicians and pharmacists, conduct studies that continuously review the effectiveness of all approved medicines. The studies demonstrate a price-effectiveness ratio that allows comparison between medicines for the same treatment and includes late effects for consumers and the environment in the price.

5.10 Pharmaceutical industry[74]

The pharmaceutical industry consists of all companies that manufacture medicines and other products used in health care. All medical devices are subject to requirements that ensure

---

73 §237,2a,2b,2d Protection of health and the environment: BV Art. 118, §238,1 Alternative medicine: BV Art. 118a
74 §236,3 Health care: KV Art.41, §239,2d,2e Research on humans: BV Art. 118b, §241,3 Transplantation medicine: BV Art. 119a

their safety and reliability. The Company Auditing Agency's health auditors are responsible for the regular auditing of pharmaceutical companies, their production methods and products. They are supported by the technical auditors when examining technical processes and products, and also by the innovation auditors when approving new medical devices.

In the production of active substances for medicines, the requirement is to use herbal active substances if possible, if they are better tolerated. Otherwise, the above requirements for medicines apply. Artificially produced organs are also considered medical devices that may be traded as usual. The requirement is that organs may not be grown in an organism that has a consciousness. An exception is the removal of organs from farm animals that are slaughtered or euthanised anyway. In the production of drugs, the pharmaceutical industry must adhere to the purity law, research long-term effects and try to produce drugs with the same effect but fewer harmful side effects.

Further requirements are of a political nature and concern the prices, quantities and novelty of medical devices. The requirements serve to keep the prices for medical devices as low as possible while maintaining the highest possible quality.

5.10.1 Pharmaceutical industry in the economic forms

Anyone who wants to start or run a pharmaceutical company has to decide in which economic form. Pharmaceutical companies in the Barter Economy are farmers, animal breeders and gardeners who breed animals and plants that are used in natural medicine procedures. They form working partnerships with pharmacists who produce medicines from them. Other medical products are produced by local handicraft enterprises on the orders of the physicians.

In Planned Economy, mainly natural remedies are used because the animal and plant raw materials for them can be cultivated in the Social Villages and processed in factories. Chemical products are produced in Social Villages with a focus on chemical industry. Other medical products are produced by Planned Enterprises.[75] All natural medicines developed in the Barter Economy and Planned Economy are in the public domain and are made available free of charge to the world population in the Knowledge Directory.

The Social Market Economy pharmaceutical industry is Non-profit. It uses its profits for research and price reduction. The state health insurance companies conclude fixed supply contracts with Social Market Economy pharmaceutical companies.

The Free Market Economy's pharmaceutical industry consists mainly of large international groups that only have to comply with the general requirements, but are not given any other economic requirements.

5.10.2 Research in the pharmaceutical industry

The pharmaceutical industry is obliged to invest a minimum share of its annual profits in research and development. This share is 5% before deduction of taxes. The companies can decide for themselves whether they want to conduct research independently or invest the money in research projects for new medical products in the Research Cost Fund, which they can choose themselves or commission.[76]

New medical products can be patented for 15 years to allow higher prices during this time and thus make research more attractive. After the patent period expires, the contents become public domain and can be imitated by other manufacturers. For medicines, these are So-called generics.

When researching new medicines and drugs, the innovation auditors of the Company Auditing Agency are the point of contact for pharmaceutical companies that establish cooperations with physicians, clinics and colleges in order to make studies possible. The pharmaceutical industry can also carry out its research and development independently, but must adhere to the same obligations as physicians in medical research. These obligations regulate in particular the handling

---

75 Ministry of Planned Economy - 11.1 Specialisation at the location, 10.5 Planned Enterprise
76 Ministry of Innovation - 5.3.1 Research Cost Fund

of persons participating in studies, So-called test persons. Experiments with animals and plants are permitted if they are unavoidable and the procedure does not assume torturous proportions.

5.10.3 Trade in medical products

In order to achieve uniformly low prices throughout the country, the Health Agency offers all physicians and pharmacists the opportunity to place collective orders for medical products via an online shop in the Health Directory. If users cannot find a desired product in the online shop, they can put it on a wish list. As soon as a sufficient number of users register their interest in buying and indicate their desired quantities, the Health Agency enters into negotiations with the manufacturers and makes the interested parties a price offer. If they accept the offer, the products are listed in the online shop. Users can also set up standing orders in the online shop, which guarantees them regular deliveries of the desired quantity at a fixed price. New medical products from the pharmaceutical industry are automatically displayed to the appropriate users as news in the online shop and are available from then on. The Health Agency conducts the price negotiations and handles the trade and logistics between the pharmaceutical industry, physicians and pharmacists. Physicians and pharmacists are free to use other trade channels to obtain medical products.

5.10.4 Pharmaceutical industry association

The pharmaceutical industry association ensures cooperation between manufacturers, the Health Agency, users of medical products and consumers of medicines and drugs. This is to determine the demand appropriately in order to avoid overproduction and shortages. In addition, physicians, physician assistants, pharmacists and patients are to express their satisfaction with the medical products and their effectiveness via the Health Directory. The task of the pharmaceutical industry association is to collect and process this information with the help of the Health Directory and to forward it to its members. In this way, the pharmaceutical industry can pursue a customer-friendly consumer policy and the Health Agency can, if necessary, intervene and regulate the pharmaceutical industry more strongly.

Particularly in times of the emergence of a new disease or an unexpected environmental catastrophe, the Health Agency can temporarily intervene in economic freedom and use the pharmaceutical industry. The pharmaceutical industry association then has the task of ensuring among its members that production is switched as quickly as possible to medical products that are needed en masse and that research is carried out into suitable testing options, medicines and vaccines.

5.11 Drugs[77]

All drugs are legal. They have always served the humans for their well-being. On the one hand, this fights organised crime and on the other hand, it increases the health of the users and creates a fair compensation of costs through the Addictive drugs Health Insurance. Drugs are treated in the same way as medicines with regard to the requirements for production and import. Purity regulations apply to production, further processing and administration. Pharmaceutical companies research how it is possible to achieve the same effect with less damage to the body. Companies producing drugs must invest 5% of their profits in this research and development.

Sale is authorised from the age of majority. Pharmacists are the first place where drugs can be bought. This means that anyone who wants to buy a drug for the first time must go to a pharmacy. After that, the catering trade and the retail trade are also authorised to sell drugs, but they must record the sale on the consumer's Health Card.

During the initial consultation, the pharmacist informs the purchaser about the optimal dosage for his or her body type and at what level of consumption a dependency sets in that leads to addiction. This information is generated using the

---

77§221,1 Drugs: BV Art. 105, §237,2a,2d Protection of health and the environment: BV Art. 118

data on the Health Card and the results of studies by the pharmaceutical industry and the Addictive drugs Health Insurance. The Health Card is also used to check whether there are risks, side effects and dangers of addiction due to the state of health, previous illnesses or due to mixed consumption. In case of doubt, the pharmacist must send the purchaser to the physician to confirm or refute possible risks through examinations. All treatment costs for the prevention of addiction and addictive diseases by pharmacists and physicians are covered by the Addictive drugs Health Insurance.

5.11.1 Limit

Each Health Card has a limit for drugs for addiction prevention. The limit is set individually for each drug user based on the personal information on the Health Card and the studies of the health auditors and the Addictive drugs Health Insurance. The limit sets a daily, weekly or monthly amount for harmless drug use. Once the limit is reached, the drug user must first see a physician who will examine him or her. The examination is to show whether the excessive drug use is damaging the client so that there is an increased risk of illness. If the risk is increased, the price of the drug that makes the client ill increases for that client. After a visit to the physician, the limit is adjusted if necessary and reset to zero. In this way, regular preventive check-ups are enforced, which prevent the drug user from becoming addicted or accompany him in it, ensure a fair cost contribution to the Addictive drugs Health Insurance and also serve the pharmaceutical industry as a long-term study to make drugs even more harmless.

5.11.2 Purity law[78]

The purity law for beer is extended to all known drugs. Pharmaceutical companies test all drugs and identify psychoactive ingredients, balancing concomitants and unnecessary impurities. Drugs on a natural basis, such as

---

[78]§221.2 Drugs

alcohol, tobacco, marijuana, opium or cocaine, must reach the consumer as naturally as possible. Additives are only permitted if they facilitate dosage, enable consumption and have no harmful effects. Breeding and crossing with different active substances and accompanying substances are possible. The natural original forms from which the cultivars have emerged must also remain available. Chemical drugs such as lysergic acid diethylamide from ergot, heroin from opium poppy or psilocybin from mushrooms should be available on a plant and chemical basis if possible. Consumers decide on the basis of their personal tolerance. Studies investigate health safety or the costs of treatment. The Company Auditing Agency's health auditors check in their own laboratories whether new, imported or domestically produced drugs comply with the purity requirement. New drugs have to go through a licensing procedure, like medicines, and are given a purity requirement tailored to them.

5.11.3 Drug card

Each time drugs are purchased, the Health Card must be used to verify age, register the purchase ensuring contribution to the Addictive drugs Health Insurance, and provide warnings for excessive or mixed drug use. For this purpose, the Addictive drugs Health Insurance is developing a suitable device in cooperation with the People's Innovation Company[79] Intranet[80] . Pharmacists and restaurateurs must be equipped with this device. It is able to measure, via data retrieval from the Health Directory and Health Card, what drug was purchased, in what quantity, over what period of time, and the contribution to the Addictive drugs Health Insurance. It automatically indicates to vendors when an excessive use warning is appropriate. Food service vendors are free to continue serving overusers or not. Drug users can access data on their consumption history through their People's Computer in the Health Directory. This data may only be used for medical purposes and is subject to confidentiality.

79 Ministry of Innovation - 10 People's Innovation Company
80 Ministry of Digital Affairs - 13 People's Innovation Company Intranet

Physicians who treat drug users must consider the side effects and interactions of the drugs in the case of certain medicines or treatment methods and measure their influence on the diagnosis. The influence of drug use on the diagnosis results in the billing of the treatment via the Addictive drugs Health Insurance. In an emergency, physicians can detect overdoses more quickly and treat them accordingly.

5.11.4 Drug research

For all drugs, voluntary long-term users are examined. The short- and long-term studies are to show how and where drugs cause damage and where they do not. In particular, drug users who are "stuck on a trip", i.e. who continue to show the mentally altered attitude without additional revenues, are also examined. The aim is to research how this effect can be avoided or used to treat chronically traumatised or depressed patients. Drug research is closely linked to medical research in order to test uses in the respective other area of application or to identify interactions with diseases or other medicines and to examine their safety.

5.12 Health insurance companies[81]

The Ministry of Health operates state health insurance funds and enables the operation of private health insurance funds in the Free Market Economy. Through the three state health insurance funds, the aim is to ensure that as much money as possible that is paid into the health insurance fund also reaches the persons who treat patients and make them healthy. All administrative tasks will be digitalised as much as possible, eliminating costs for clerks' salaries, managers and buildings. While the General Health Insurance is a health insurance for general diseases and injuries, the Addictive drugs Health Insurance only covers preventive measures for addiction, treatment of addictive diseases and consequential damages

---

81 §45.1b Welfare state: BV Art.41, §235.1 Health and accident insurance: BV Art. 117, §236.10 Health care

of drug use. Immortality Health Insurance only covers life-sustaining measures in the last three months of life. Private health insurance companies can also cover other treatments that are not covered by the state health insurance companies. All health insurance companies offer health prevention options and treatments to keep their insured as healthy as possible.

5.12.1 Insurance benefits in the economic forms

Compulsory insurance in a health insurance fund differs between economic forms. The only compulsory insurance is the Addictive drugs Health Insurance, whose premiums are paid through price surcharges on addictive drugs. The General Health Insurance is the general compulsory insurance in the Barter Economy, Barter Economy and Social Market Economy, paid for by business taxes, in-kind contributions or labour services. Immortality Health Insurance is a voluntary supplementary insurance, regardless of the economic form from which one derives one's main income.

Citizens who earn their main income in the Free Market Economy are not required to have health insurance at all, but may be members of the General Health Insurance and the Immortality Health Insurance, or of a private health, care or accident insurance scheme.

Nationals who need health care but do not have health insurance and do not have enough money for treatment can get treatment at a Social Village health centre. To receive such benefits, they must leave the Free Market Economy and live and work in the Planned Economy until the costs incurred have been developed, either through working hours or through business taxes in the luxury supply work area.

In the Barter Economy, all physicians and medical assistants at the hospital must receive food and clean clothes and medical products through the patients. Those who have been treated in the hospital are obliged to do so for a certain period of time, depending on the cost of the treatment, once they are well again. The equipment for treatments is the discarded goods of the state and private medical practices and hospitals. The medicines used are either natural remedies grown in the

Barter Economy or generic drugs. Thus, the cost of health care is largely borne by the Barter Economy and the rest is provided from tax revenues generated by the Barter Economy. External financing is excluded. In case of doubt, the medical care must support fewer services.

In Planned Economy, health care is considered part of the basic supply and is provided by the labour input of all Social Villagers. Medical products are generic drugs, old and repaired discarded devices from private and state medical practices, hospitals and university clinics or own productions from Planned Enterprises. Imports of missing medical products are procured through the General Health Insurance and paid for through business taxes.

5.12.2 General Health Insurance[82]

The General Health Insurance is a state health insurance that covers all Medical Fee Schedule treatment, whether due to illness or accident. As another voluntary option, insured persons can also take out long-term care insurance.

In the Social Market Economy there is a legal obligation to be insured with the General Health Insurance. Companies must contribute 15% of the remuneration paid to employees and owners to the health insurance fund. The percentage of the contribution rate depends on the costs incurred by the members.

In the Free Market Economy, the insurance is available with the General Health Insurance with a monthly premium that is adjusted to the health status of the insured person. In the Free Market Economy, there is also an excess of 10%, up to a maximum of 1000 Dollars. The excess is to be paid directly at the time of treatment or on account. The remaining amount is transferred to the physician by the General Health Insurance at the end of the month.

If the General Health Insurance's reserves are not sufficient, a fixed amount is charged for the most expensive patients. The limit at which one belongs to the most expensive patients and how high the fixed amount is depends on the General

82§235.3 Health and accident insurance

Health Insurance's cash balance. By disclosing the budget, insured persons are entitled to vote on an adjustment of the contributions for the coming year in the course of the annual budget vote. The Minister of Health is responsible for premium adjustments during the year.

5.12.2.1 Accident insurance[83]

Accident insurance is used for the prevention of accidents, rescue measures, medical treatment and compensation after accidents. It is part of the General Health Insurance. Accident insurance pays for accident prevention measures resulting from a workplace safety audit by the Company Auditing Agency's health auditors. If accidents at work or occupational diseases do occur that render an employee unable to work, accident insurance continues to pay the employee's wages until the employee's pension is paid. The accident insurance scheme democratically votes with all contributors on which benefits from the seventh social security code[84] should be covered. Furthermore, accident insurance is additionally a liability insurance that covers costs for damage that was not caused by gross negligence.

5.12.3 Addictive drugs Health Insurance[85]

The Addictive drugs Health Insurance is a compulsory insurance intended for planned harmful acts. It thus protects other insured persons who do not expose themselves to such health hazards by covering health care costs incurred by the Addictive drugs Health Insurance. The Addictive drugs Health Insurance also finances disability, care and pension insurance. Addicted persons and addicted pensioners can move into the Social Village at any time if they have become incapacitated or in need of care due to addictive substances. The revenues of the Addictive drugs Health Insurance are then paid out as

83 §235.3 Health and accident insurance
84 http://www.gesetze-im-internet.de/sgb_7/
85 §221.3 Drugs: BV Art. 105, §222,3 Money games: BV Art. 106, §236,3 Health care: KV Art.41, §235,2 Health and Accident Insurance

a subsidy to the Planned Economy because the Social Villages provide a treatment service. Physicians and pharmacists are obliged to inform patients whose treatments they bill via the Addictive drugs Health Insurance about their options for preventive measures against addiction.

All intoxicants, such as heroin, marijuana, nicotine, alcohol or caffeine, all food additives that increase consumption, trigger cravings or drive blood sugar levels to extremes, such as simple sugar or wheat flour without the whole grain, are considered hazardous to health. In the same way, tattoo studios have to pay a contribution per tattoo, which is higher the larger the tattooed area of a human is. The percentage of a human's skin surface area is taken as the assessment threshold for how much the toxins in the ink will damage the liver over the course of a lifetime. Casinos and operators of slot machines must pay 75% of gross gaming revenue to the Addictive drugs Health Insurance. For all consumer goods that are harmful to health, a price surcharge is levied on the good or service, which is paid to the Addictive drugs Health Insurance as a contribution.

Extreme sports with a high risk of injury are also affected. Those who practise these sports must do so in a club that pays the health insurance contribution through its membership fees, or at a corresponding event, the organiser must collect the contributions through the entrance fees and pay them to the Addictive drugs Health Insurance. If an extreme athlete cannot or does not want to be a member of any club, he/she must pay the treatment costs himself/herself. In the case of brawls, the participants must visit the People's Protection Service before or after the brawl if injuries require medical treatment so that the appropriate contribution can be paid through the body injury billing device.[86]

The Addictive drugs Health Insurance is the only health insurance scheme that draws its contributions from all four economic forms. Manufacturers have to pay the contributions for each product they put into circulation as soon as they deliver it. For example, Mc Donalds, Phillip Morris and Bayer pay the contributions as soon as they reach their domestic customers. If goods spoil, the contribution is not refunded.

86Ministry of Security - 6.1.4 Tools

The contribution is applied to each unit circulating inland, such as a hamburger receives a 20 cent surcharge, as does a cigarette, 0.33 litre of beer or 0.1 gram of marijuana. Prices are adjusted for diagnosed diseases and their treatment costs. Depending on how many consumers an addictive substance makes ill, the price surcharge will be higher or lower. Should an addictive substance be produced in such a wholesome way or should the consumers comply with their limit, the price surcharges for this addictive substance can be lowered.

5.12.4 Immortality Health Insurance[87]

Health care services provided in the last three months of life are billed through Immortality Health Insurance. If someone has a terminal illness or injury and the remaining life expectancy is less than three months, life support will only be provided by all currently available means if this health insurance was additionally taken out before the diagnosis. Your contribution is based on the current number of patients in a pay-as-you-go system. This health insurance is a supplementary insurance that can be taken out by all citizens who are able to pay for it. The contributions increase when there are many insured people undergoing treatment and decrease when there are fewer. The Immortality Health Insurance creates a market for life-prolonging treatments that is worth researching. The research results will first benefit the insured when they are treated with them. At the same time, or after the patent expires, all humans benefit from the new state of science and technology. Because researchers depend on data and test persons, there are benefits. Those who release all their data from the Health Directory and their Health Card for research purposes receive a bonus of 10% lower contributions. Those who indicate in their living will that they may be used as a test patient or who donate their body to research after their death can receive a further 10% discount on their contributions. For test patients, treatment is free if the risk of damage or failure is high.

87§235.2 Health and accident insurance

5.12.5 Health insurance association

All private and state health insurance funds are united in this association. Its task is to make an overview of the contributions of all patients possible. Here, it is particularly important for the insured to be able to switch easily between different economic forms. In the Free Market Economy, it is not necessary to have health insurance, but it is important for the Ministry of Health to know how many citizens do not have health insurance. The Health Insurance Association collects this data and forwards it to the Health Agency every year. The Health Agency can also request the data at another time. The Health Insurance Fund Association represents the health insurance funds on committees and ensures that the health insurance funds are informed of new requirements from the Ministry of Health.

The health insurance association compiles the cash balances of all insurance companies. In this way, premium adjustments can be made for individual or all insured persons. Through the association, all health insurance companies have access to a patient's data, provided he or she wants to take out insurance with them. However, the patient data only includes the costs of treatment and medication and the frequency of doctor visits, but not the diagnoses or Medical Fee Schedule billing numbers. The Company Auditing Agency's health auditors check this data set every 2 years directly with the attending physician and the entries in the Health Directory with their admission to all patient data.

6 Health prevention[88]

The Ministry of Health pursues a policy of health prevention that enables the humans in the country to exercise in a healthy environment and to eat healthily through it. Every citizen can take care of his or her health through a balanced diet and sufficient exercise. In addition to the personal responsibility for exercise and nutrition, as well as their independent execution, the Ministry of Health provides the legal framework. In order to be able to keep healthy, requirements for the safety of food

---

88§45.1b Welfare state: BV Art.41

and products are drawn up and audited. In order to keep future generations healthy, requirements and measures for a circular economy, sustainable use of nature and environmental protection are drawn up and checked.

6.1 Nutrition

Nutrition is primarily the responsibility of a private individual. The Ministry of Labour supports healthy nutrition through a food traffic light and healthy food production without harmful residues in the food.[89] The Ministry of Education ensures through its educational institutions that everyone knows how to eat healthily[90], and that nutrition science is kept up to date. The Ministry of Infrastructure supports fresh free healthy food close to home by planting edible plants on public land.[91] The Ministry of Health verifies the conditions of edibility and safety of these public foods through soil sampling and fruit sampling. As a prerequisite, the traffic along these areas must be free of pollutants.

Health care professionals are employed to help citizens make healthy dietary choices. Since a healthy diet is different for each human organism and according to age, physicians are responsible for the examination and record personal physical characteristics in the Health Directory every 10 years. Citizens can use this data for their shopping and nutrition. Via an additional application in the Health Directory, every citizen can access his or her data record. By scanning or photographing the barcode of food with their camera in the People's Computer and manually selecting appropriate proposals from a list, food data can be retrieved from the Food Directory[92]. In addition, retailers offer cash register receipts that contain a barcode with data on the food purchased for 24 hours.

With these data sets, an algorithm can suggest the healthiest diet for each person. The Institute of Environmental Medicine, in cooperation with physicians, researches which processing measures and composition of foods are related to which

89 Ministry of Labour - 17.7.2 Food traffic light, 19 Agriculture
90 Ministry of Education - 9.15.1.5 School subject in the ninth learning year: Nutrition
91 Ministry of Infrastructure - 4.3.2 Agricultural land
92 Ministry of Labour - 19.13 Food Directory

consumption habits and diets are beneficial or harmful.

In the case of communal catering, on the other hand, the requirements are stronger than for individual catering, because individuals have less influence here. Suppliers of communal catering have to adjust their meals to their regular clients. To do this, all clients can share their healthy eating record from the Health Directory with the mass catering supplier, who retrieves the data through the company's profile in the Labour Directory. Through this companion application, ordering processes, cooking recipes and workflows can be automatically adapted to the clients' requirements.

6.1.1 Guidelines for a healthy diet

The Ministry of Health, in cooperation with the Ministry of Labour, ensures that the food available in the country is produced in such a way that it does as little damage to the body as possible. Manufacturers who do not want to do without this have to pay price surcharges as contributions to the Addictive drugs Health Insurance. The health auditors monitor compliance with the following requirements and control them before first marketing and thereafter as part of their regular audits of the company.

Food must be free of pathogens such as viruses, bacteria, fungi, pests or toxins. The Institute of Environmental Medicine sets limit values that apply to products, humans, animals, plants, water, air and soil. In the course of the medical examinations, patients are also tested to see whether the limit values are complied with. The costs for these additional examinations are borne by the Company Auditing Agency and invoiced to the affected companies in the course of an audit.

If a product is found to be of dubiousness during the initial testing, long-term studies over 5 years must be proven. At least 1000 test persons are examined by three different state colleges, which must include at least one university hospital. A re-screening is foreseen every 15 years. After 5 years without any complaints, the food is allowed to be sold in the trade. All customers are asked to participate in the study at the time of purchase and to regularly indicate when and how often they consume the product. This will now also appear in the patient's file with the physician, who is entitled to carry out and charge for a prescribed annual examination. The costs for this must be borne by the manufacturing or importing company.

The health auditors determine which food traffic light category the food falls into during their initial assessment. If a food with a red label triggers health complaints, a price surcharge is initiated for the contribution to the Addictive drugs Health Insurance. The price mark-up must be indicated on the price label. This allows customers to see whether the price mark-up is high and whether this product has already made many humans ill accordingly.

6.2 Exercise[93]

For sporting activities on land, in water and in the air, the Ministry of Health, in cooperation with the Ministry of Infrastructure, operates areas for sporting activities for the population.[94] These include, for example, trim trails, running tracks, bicycle circuits, climbing trees and climbing facades on bridges or state buildings, as well as entry and exit points on rivers, lakes and coastal areas where all kinds of water sports may be practised.

Safety precautions are attached to the climbing trees and facades. At the top, a shock absorber is connected to a fall chain that climbers can hook onto. It is designed to prevent impact with the ground and cushion the fall. The chains extend two metres above the ground. At the end of them are carabiners that you can hook into either your belt or a climbing harness. Safety precautions for swimmers are buoy strings in the river, similar to lane boundaries in swimming pools. They are placed in places with strong currents or close shipping traffic. The buoy strings are stretched between the green and red buoys. This makes it obvious which lane is for motorised watercraft. On the outer sides, up to the shore, there is space for swimmers and rowers. If the current pushes you away or ships would pull swimmers into the middle of the river with their suction, you

93§184.2 Promotion of music, sport, film, culture and art: BV Art.68
94Ministry of Infrastructure - 4.6 Leisure

can hold on to the buoys.

Sports clubs can apply to the Building Office for space for their sports facilities and offer their services to educational institutions. The health auditors check the devices and training methods as part of their regular inspection.

Companies whose executives carry out work that involves little or moderate movement must offer physical activity breaks and, from a size of 50 employees, company sports. These occupational health and safety measures are adapted to the duty rosters and physical stress zones by the health auditors in terms of time and method. Part of the audit is a company medical examination of physical fitness.

6.3 Food safety[95]

The ministries of labour and economy regulate the production of food. The Ministry of Health ensures laws that guarantee the health safety of food. The Ministry of Health is responsible for legislation in food law that affects health. The Institute for Medicines and Foodstuffs, together with the Ministry of Labour, develops regulations on the labelling of origin, quality, production method and processing methods for foodstuffs.[96]

This includes labelling through a food traffic light and ingredient list that can be voted on their personal health status through the Food Directory and the Health Directory for consumers.[97]

The origin of a food product must be traceable for traders and consumers. The food chain extends from raw materials and ingredients to the final product with names and addresses of all companies involved.[98]

The quality must meet the requirements for the safety of the food chain. Cold chains must not be interrupted, residues and contaminants must not reach or enter the food during production, further processing, transport or trade. It must be shielded by suitable packaging and production methods.

95 §237.2a Protection of health and the environment: BV Art. 118, §220.3d Agriculture: BV Art. 104
96 Ministry of Labour - 17.7 Consumer Information Standards
97 Ministry of Labour - 17.7.2 Food traffic light, 19.13 Food Directory
98 Ministry of Labour - 17.7.3 Origin display

Particular attention is paid to meat hygiene in order to prevent the spread of animal diseases to other animals or to humans. The Ministry of Labour issues further requirements for food quality.[99]

Production methods must be sustainable and protect the environment. Raw materials must not be used beyond what is necessary so that future generations will continue to have the same or greater amount of raw materials available. Environmental protection is guaranteed if production is embedded in a circular economy and does not release pollutants. The Ministry of Labour issues the necessary requirements for the food industry[100], which also affect processing methods.

The industry's processing methods for food, medicine and consumer goods must meet food safety standards. This includes all objects that are absorbed into the body or come into contact with the body or food and medicines, So-called food contact materials. During processing, no residues of pharmacologically active or toxic substances may be produced in food and no additives that are hazardous to health may be added.

In the case of food and medicines, a best-before date must be indicated on the product until which health safety is guaranteed under the specified storage conditions. The health auditors check this date at the time of authorisation to see if it is appropriate and during their regular audits to see if it is adhered to.

The health auditors of the Company Auditing Agency are responsible for food monitoring. They check compliance with the regulations on labelling of origin, quality, production method and processing methods, thus ensuring sufficient food hygiene and consumer health protection. In the event of violations, the health auditors provide detection, evidence gathering and, in cooperation with the Health Agency, crisis management. Crisis management eliminates the causes and consequences of the violations. Health prevention also includes nutritional prevention, for which the Ministry of Health is responsible and establishes emergency reserves in cooperation

99 Ministry of Labour - 19.5 Food quality
100 Ministry of Labour - 19.8 Food industry

with the Ministry of Security.[101] The health auditors verify the sufficiency of reserves and their proper storage.

6.4 Product safety[102]

The Ministry of Health regulates the handling of products, pollutants, pollution, genetically modified genetic material, noise pollution and radiation that can endanger the health of humans and the environment in product safety law. This applies in particular to products of the biotechnological, chemical and pharmaceutical industries as well as the energy, transport and data transmission industries. Each industry bears an industry-specific product responsibility adapted to it. The product safety standards ensure safety for consumers' health or explicitly warn of health hazards emanating from a product and provide for shielded storage or use.

Products must have a best-before date on the product until which it is safe for the human and natural environment under certain weather conditions. The health auditors check this date at the time of authorisation to see if it is appropriate and in their regular audits to see if it is adhered to.

Company Auditing Agency for Health and Technology auditors test all products before they are approved for the domestic market and award seals of approval[103] for successfully tested products. Companies that use or sell dangerous products are regularly audited for compliance with the standards, sometimes unannounced or undercover.

Products using genetic engineering are subject to bioethics, which the Minister of Health determines in a committee with the people. This is to avoid ethically questionable late effects or abuses or to do so with the consent of the people.

Products sourced from abroad must also comply with the requirements of the ministries of health and labour. If this is violated abroad, the domestic-based company will be brought before a domestic court by the responsible domestic

---

101 Ministry of Security - 5.7 Disaster management
102 §237,2a,2c Protection of health and the environment: BV Art. 118,
§242,1 Genetic engineering in the non-human sector: BV Art. 120
103 Ministry of Labour - 17.7.4 Seal of approval

investigating authorities of the Company Auditing Agency, police and public prosecutors.

6.5 Sustainable use of nature[104]

The Ministry of Health is responsible for the sustainable use of nature in the country. It takes appropriate requirements and measures to preserve the health of humans, animals, plants and their habitats for future generations. Organisms, chemicals and other objects that endanger health are prohibited or their handling is regulated by law. In the event of accidents, diseases or overloads that endanger the health of nature, a crisis centre is set up at the Health Agency, which determines the measures to be taken and monitors their timely implementation in cooperation with the health auditors.

Sustainable use of nature is ensured when nature is given sufficient time and space to regenerate from human intervention, protected areas provide nature with sufficient retreats, plants and animals are protected from abuse and extinction, agriculture enriches the ecosystem and when the global ecosystem is protected from uncontrolled genetic modification.

6.5.1 Sustainability[105]

Sustainability here means that nature may only be used by humans to the extent that it is able to grow back sufficiently. Natural regrowth is considered to be capable of renewal, and renewal is complete when the state prior to the claim has been restored. Anticipation of future generations is prohibited. For example, a new tree must be planted for a felled tree, which in turn may not be felled until it has reached the same size as its predecessor. If humans want to cut down more trees than are currently growing back and simply plant additional trees, only the additionally planted trees may be used and no existing

---

104§191,4 Nature and homeland protection: BV Art. 78, §220,3e
Agriculture: BV Art. 104, §237,1,2a Protection of health and environment: BV Art. 118
105§189.2 Sustainability, §190.2 Environmental protection: KV Art.31

trees. Sufficient renewal capacity must first be established before an ecosystem can be put under additional strain. This is to ensure that future generations have as much or more at their disposal as the current generation and to prevent a decline in living standards. The exploitation of nature beyond its renewal capacity is considered negligent physical injury to the following generation. The spreading of deadly pollutants that accumulate in nature is considered negligent homicide of the following generation.

Only renewable raw materials may be used, and only to a limited extent. This limit is set by nature with its local conditions. For example, bamboo cannot grow at all or only slowly in a barren polar region, whereas it can grow very quickly in subtropical regions. If humans want to use bamboo, it must be ensured that no more bamboo is felled than can grow back. Accordingly, in subtropical regions, humans are likely to use more bamboo. These restrictions apply regionally. They can also apply internationally if global production does not exceed global natural growth and suitable transport options exist to all regions.

6.5.2 Nature reserves[106]

Nature reserves are areas where nature is protected from human interference. The Health Agency selects primeval nature areas in the country and proposes to the Minister of Health that these areas be protected with restricted or prohibited human use. Nature reserves are divided into nature parks, where no human use is allowed at all, and landscape, bird and water protection areas, where human use is restricted. Restrictions are placed on agriculture and the construction of transport routes, commercial and residential buildings. The restriction of such infrastructural interventions is adapted to the landscape, bird or water protection object.

Forests are protected by landscape conservation areas. The forestry use of the forest can be fully or partially restricted. The partial restriction means that trees may only be felled and

---

106§190,5 Environmental protection: KV Art.31, §193,2 Forest: BV Art. 77, §191,4,5 Nature and homeland protection: BV Art. 78

planted along existing forest paths, while 5 metres away from the forest paths the forest ecosystem itself takes care of the seeding and decomposition of deadwood.

Water bodies and zones around sources and storage facilities of drinking water are protected by water protection areas. The use of rivers, lakes and coastal areas for fishing, as transport routes or for water sports may be restricted in whole or in part. Restricted use may specify fishing quotas and fishing areas for fishermen and prohibit certain means of transport and water sports. Fishing, transport and water sports are generally not permitted in the vicinity of drinking water resources. Exceptions may apply if only fully biodegradable items are used.

Pristine natural areas are zones in the long landscape where rare species and breeds of animals and plants occur that are unique to an ecosystem. If species are threatened with extinction, a nature park must be created for them. Use by humans is fundamentally excluded there. Humans visiting a nature park are only allowed to move along designated paths. Nature parks enable biodiversity because they provide refuges from which diverse species and breeds of plants and animals can spread into the surrounding countryside. Biodiversity means the variety of breeds, species and ecosystems. Ecosystems here mean landscapes that provide different habitats for species that have adapted to them, such as mountains, coasts, forests, moors or lowlands.

6.5.3 Animal and plant protection[107]

The Ministry of Health is responsible for the protection of animals and plants. Plants are considered protected if they are allowed to grow in a manner appropriate to their species. Animals are considered protected if they are housed, fed, sanitised and medically cared for in a manner appropriate to their species. The wanton torture of animals is prohibited. No consideration is given to religious concerns in animal protection. Entrepreneurs who offer animal trade and transport must keep and care for animals in a manner appropriate to

107 §194 Animal welfare: BV Art. 80

their species while they are in their care.

In cooperation with Customs, veterinarians and plant doctors check the import of animals and plants and confirm their health. Sick animals and plants or animals and plants that could disturb the local ecosystem may not be brought into the country. The Health Agency determines the animal and plant species affected.

6.5.3.1 Plant health

Healthy plants are the basis for healthy animals and humans because they serve them as a source of food and a filtering system for waste gases and excretions. The Health Agency makes requirements to ensure plant health, which is checked by health auditors in companies and state enterprises. On public land, the Ministry of Infrastructure is responsible for ensuring plant health.[108] Healthy plants live in soils that provide them with sufficient nutrients and are free of toxins that would not allow any plant to survive there. Soil polluted with certain contaminants or poor in nutrients can be improved by growing certain plants. The Health Agency can order the planting of such plants to improve soil quality, which increases overall plant health. For the protection of bees and insects, fertilising or protecting plants with substances that are harmful to these animals is prohibited. The Health Agency excludes affected substances from trade.

6.5.3.2 Feed and fertiliser

Feed safety is about ensuring plant health on the one hand and animal health on the other. Plant fertilisers must not be contaminated with substances that are harmful to the animals to be fed. Animal feed must not be contaminated with toxins and pathogens. The feeding of animals to animals or humans is only permissible if the animals are free of diseases and medicines at the time of death. This is to prevent the transmission of pathogens between different animal species

---

108 Ministry of Infrastructure - 4.3.2 Agricultural land

or humans. It is also intended to prevent the education of pathogens resistant to a medicine and the transfer of medicine residues in the food chain.

6.5.3.3 Killing of animals

Wild animals can roam freely in the wild and are killed by hunters if they pose a danger to humans or are in excessive numbers due to a lack of natural predators. The Health Agency monitors wild animal populations and can release them for shooting.

Pets must belong to a human who keeps and cares for them in a manner appropriate to their species. Pets may be medically treated and killed by veterinarians at the request of the owner. Farm animals must belong to a company that provides species-appropriate husbandry and care. They may be killed by veterinarians, researchers or butchers if the entrepreneur or a responsible employee requests it. The killing of animals must be carried out free of pain and stress for the animals. Farmed animals for meat processing must not be given toxic substances to kill them. Farm animals for research must not be unnecessarily tortured. Animal experiments and procedures on live animals must be carried out using current anaesthetics, unless this makes the research project impossible. The health auditors observe these requirements in their examination of research projects involving animal experiments. The Health Agency sets the requirements for species-appropriate killing, which are checked by the health auditors at veterinarians, research and slaughter facilities.

6.5.3.4 Audit

Compliance with these requirements is checked on the one hand by the health auditors during their regular company audits and on the other hand by veterinarians during their examinations. Veterinarians are only obliged to administer veterinary medicines if these medicines do not also serve humans and thus resistant pathogens can arise. If veterinarians diagnose transmissible diseases in animals, they must report these incidents to the Health Agency. The Health Agency monitors incidents and, in the event of a spreading animal disease, may order the isolation and killing of animals to contain the disease.

6.5.4 Marine protection

International water management is regulated by all states, which undertake to comply with the requirements because the majority of their peoples have spoken out in favour of them. Shipping companies are obliged to leave all cargo on board all their ships and not to dispose of anything in the oceans except non-toxic treated wastewater.

The Ministry of Health issues these rules for all vessels entering its territorial waters or domestic ports. The Ministry of Health, in cooperation with the Ministry of Foreign Affairs, is committed to strengthening international cooperation for the protection of the world's oceans and international river basins in order to establish uniform requirements and implement joint measures.

All companies involved in the production of plastic and plastic articles must pay for the cleaning of the oceans from plastic waste. The use of plastic in the oceans is prohibited. All plastics that can come into contact with seawater and be lost in it must be made of biodegradable plastic that must have degraded in seawater within 2 years. Suitable protection against high and low tides will be instituted in coastal areas. Suitable reefs will be established in cooperation with the Ministry of Infrastructure through the targeted settlement of shells and corals.

6.5.5 Agriculture[109]

The Ministry of Labour is responsible for agriculture. The Ministry of Health issues the necessary requirements for health protection. This includes landscape maintenance of

---

109§195 Fishing and hunting: BV Art. 79, §220,3e,4 Agriculture: BV

public and agricultural land by farmers. The landscape should support the inhabitants' recreation and provide them with fresh air and moisture. Agri-environmental measures are all those requirements of the Ministry of Health through which agriculture contributes to environmental protection. These are measures such as permaculture[110] or the reduction of methane through an adapted type of feeding or the limitation of farm animals that emit excessive amounts of methane compared to other farm animals with comparable nutrient content. Farm animals that emit a lot of methane can only be kept in airtight barns after a certain number, where the methane can be filtered and converted into electricity or heat. No consideration is given to religious concerns in environmental protection. Similarly, in order to protect the environment, no fertilisers, chemicals or genetically modified substances may be used on near-natural agricultural land. In unnatural agricultural areas[111] the use of such substances is permitted as long as they cannot enter the free ecosystem. The same applies to the use of medicines for farm animals. The death of a farm animal is acceptable as long as it allows medicines to remain effective for humans. In the case of genetically modified organisms, it must be ensured that neither seeds, pollen and plants nor animals enter the free environment during production and transport. Their transport through the environment must take place in packaging that prevents escape.

Hunting of wild animals and fishing are also part of agriculture and are subject to the same requirements. Wild animals killed by hunting or fishing must be checked by a veterinarian before being consumed by humans or animals. Wild animals may only be hunted if their population is not endangered and their population assumes an excessive size or poses a danger to humans. Overgrowth is when the population of a wild animal species increases because it has no natural enemy in the affected area and a further increase in population would endanger the other animals and plants in the ecosystem. Animal species threatened with extinction

---

Art. 104, BV Art. 197
110 Ministry of Labour - 19.8.7 Nature-based agriculture: permaculture
111 Ministry of Labour - 19.8.8 Agriculture away from nature: Indoor agribusiness

may only be hunted if they pose a danger to humans and their survival can be guaranteed in at least 2 natural parks. The Health Agency takes over the adaptation of the requirements to the individual parts of the country and ecosystems. The health auditors regularly check the agricultural companies for compliance with the requirements.

6.5.6 Genetic engineering[112]

The Ministry of Health is responsible for the legal requirements for the use of genetic engineering in the non-human sector. The use of genetic engineering can have an uncontrolled and unintended impact on the global ecosystem and damage its health. To prevent such occurrences, the Health Agency provides requirements to prevent any contact of genetically modified organisms with the environment. Germ and genetic material of animals, plants and other organisms is considered common property and cannot be protected by an industrial property right. Genetically manipulated germ and hereditary material, on the other hand, can. It loses its patent protection after 20 years and is then in the public domain. It is forbidden to make genetically modified plants seed-proof or animals capable of procreation. It is also forbidden to deprive natural plants or animals of their seed firmness or procreative capacity. If genetically modified organisms are to be approved in the free environment after successful long-term studies and simulations of propagation in the free ecosystem after 25 years at the earliest, all affected peoples must vote by a majority in favour.

The dignity of the genetically created creature is considered to be preserved if it is given the necessary animal and plant protection. The ethics committee[113] must decide on the gift of consciousness. In the event of approval, the health auditors check all subsequent procedures and report regularly. Before approval is granted, a committee must set the necessary requirements for the handling of the artificially created creature

112 §220,4 Agriculture: BV Art. 197, §242,2,3 Genetic engineering in the non-human sector: BV Art. 120
113 Ministry of State Organisation - 8.5.9 Ethics Commission

with consciousness and, in a voting, decide by a majority in favour of approval under the above requirements.

To protect genetic diversity, all animal and plant species, and if possible their breeds, are included in the gene database. Hereditary diseases are investigated and can be eradicated by genetic engineering.

6.6 Environmental protection[114]

The environment consists of animate and inanimate nature as well as humans. When we speak of environmental protection, we mean that animate and inanimate nature should be protected from human intervention so that it remains able to maintain itself in a healthy state. Environmental protection for humans means that the environment is healthy in such a way that humans can also remain healthy in it. Humans can insure themselves against the damage they do to themselves. The environment is insured by the state. The Ministry of Health and its agencies are primarily responsible for this insurance. Therefore, it issues regularisations for state and private activities to ensure that the environment is only regeneratively polluted.

The Ministry of Health is responsible for environmental protection and regulates interdepartmental principles in environmental law. This obliges all ministries and state activities, as well as private individuals and companies in the country, to provide environmental protection. Persons entering the country from abroad and companies importing goods and services must comply with environmental law. Environmental law contains all the above requirements for food, agriculture, product safety, the circular economy and the use of nature, as well as for climate protection and environmental protection.

Climate protection means protecting the Earth's temperature conditions from human influences, especially when they are unintended or out of control.

Environmental protection means the protection of air, water and soil from noise, harmful gases, liquids and solids. The aim of the Ministry of Health's requirements is to prevent this

114§190,1,3 Environmental protection: KV Art.31, BV Art.74

damage from occurring in the first place or to ensure proper disposal.

The health auditors report all their data to the Statistical Office[115] . The Health Agency uses this collection of data to continuously compile information on the state of health of the environment in statistics. Based on these statistics, the Minister of Health decides on the necessity of selective elimination of environmental damage or the initiation of structural change.

6.6.1 Environment Directory

In the Environment Directory, all environmental damage is given a profile. Environmental damage can include environmentally harmful products, services, habits, accidents, illegal waste dumping and disposal of exhaust gases, waste water and noise in the environment. All environmentally sound competing products are listed in the profile.

Every user can create a profile. For this, users document the environmental damage by photo, video or text. Locations of illegal waste dumping are also marked with a dot on the map and the coordinates. If illegal waste is regularly dumped at these locations, undercover cameras with motion sensors are installed to make it easier to track down the offenders.

The profiles serve as an exchange forum for users and affected parties to share experiences and introduce legislative initiatives to the appropriate ministry, to make proposals to the appropriate parties and their working groups, or to submit a case to News Television with a high level of user attention.[116] An algorithm correlates the profiles to indicate which companies and persons are responsible for damage discovered either domestically or elsewhere in the world. The results are automatically forwarded to the police for persons and to health auditors for companies.

Voluntary persons and disposal companies can form groups in which they gather to remove an environmental damage and then delete its profile. The health auditors also enter their

115 Ministry of Digital Affairs - 6 Statistical Office
116 Ministry of Media - 8 News Television

measurements and test results of environmental damage in the corresponding profiles and check whether the environmental damage of deleted profiles has actually been removed. Anyone who has deleted a profile without the environmental damage actually having been eliminated receives the same sentence as if they had caused the environmental damage themselves.

6.6.2 Regenerative impact

A regenerative load is given when nature is able to renew itself in such a way that the original state is restored through a circular economy, environmentally neutral disposal, effective and economical use of raw materials. Accordingly, nature may only be burdened by each human generation in such a way that by the time it is next used, it has at least reached the state it was in before it was used. Environmental conditions may improve for the next generation, but not deteriorate. A human generation is 30 years. If finite raw materials are used, another possibility must be invented within 30 years to replace the finite raw material for the following generation.

6.6.3 Environmentally neutral disposal

Environmentally neutral disposal means that after the disposal process, all residues could be deposited in the environment and would biodegrade through natural action within 30 years. However, environmentally neutral disposal also stipulates that residual substances may only be introduced into the environment in accordance with applicable requirements. Residual substances are waste, noise, waste water and exhaust gas. They are considered a harmful and nuisance impact on the environment. They cannot be avoided, but they can be reduced to the lowest possible level. The Ministry of Health sets requirements for this.
Waste must be recycled or biologically processed so that it can be immediately degraded by the natural ecosystem.[117] Hazardous waste is not degradable with the current state of

---

117Ministry of Infrastructure - 4.9.2.2 Waste recycling plants

research and must be stored in an accessible and harmless manner. The production of goods that become hazardous waste is prohibited. As soon as all contaminated sites could be disposed of in an environmentally neutral way through research and development, all current costs for hazardous waste disappear.

Industrially generated noise is avoided by all means. On the one hand, companies are bound by requirements because only new products that generate as little noise as possible are approved and old noisy products must be retrofitted or disposed of by a deadline. For example, a car door must close as quietly as possible instead of imitating the sound of a closing car door from previous years. On the other hand, research institutions are developing innovations that make as little noise as possible. For example, blades, rotor blades of turbines and the exhaust tubes at the end of them are frayed like owl feathers to move silently through the air.

Wastewater must be channelled through a sewer system into a treatment plant so that it would be drinkable by humans after it leaves the treatment plant. Exhaust gases must be filtered in such a way that humans could inhale them directly.

6.6.4 Negative environmental externalities

When persons or companies dispose of their waste, noise, wastewater or exhaust gas in the environment, they save on disposal costs, can charge lower prices and make higher profits. The effect is therefore positive for the originators. Outsiders profit neither from the low prices nor from the profits, but have to bear the costs. In economic terms, negative externalities are therefore costs that are passed on to outsiders. Legally, this is theft or expropriation. The Ministry of Health, as the insurer of the environment, is responsible for giving legal voice to the incapable animals, plants and children. Originators of negative environmental externalities are investigated and brought to justice by Company Auditing Agency auditors, Health Agency staff and police.[118] Judgments

118 Ministry of Justice - 8.11.6 Negative externalities, 8.1.3 Corporate criminal law

result in compensation payments and monetary fines. These monies are transferred to the Ministry of Health to pay for the clean-up of the pollution. If necessary, tax funds are requested in the budget and if the budget vote is positive, the clean-up is financed by tax funds until the amount of damage has been reimbursed with interest by the originator.

6.6.5 Elimination of environmental disasters

The Health Agency is responsible for identifying environmental disasters and cooperates with the health auditors for measurements and inventories. First and foremost, the originators should ensure that all environmental damage is cleaned up without leaving any residue. If responsible companies and private individuals cannot bear the costs and become insolvent, all those responsible have to go into detention to pay off the costs. If their life time is not sufficient for this, the state must pay for the remaining costs and ensure that the damage is removed without residue. The Health Agency maintains a department for the current industries that generate environmental disasters. In today's world, widespread pollution with petroleum products, incalculable amounts of radiated nuclear waste from nuclear power and poisoned mine water from mining are considered three environmental disasters affecting the country.

The International Oil Pollution Compensation Funds (IOPC)[119] is used for the disposal of past environmental damage caused by petroleum products. In addition, current petroleum products have to pay a price surcharge that is able to compensate for all the damage caused by the petroleum products sold.

A special form of waste is radioactive radiation from nuclear waste. They are so special and rare that they cannot be recycled by the usual disposal companies. The nuclear industry must provide for the construction and operation of specialised disposal companies. The safety of nuclear institutions, sufficient measures for radiation protection and nuclear waste disposal are checked by health auditors. The radiating waste

---

119https://www.iopcfunds.org/

of nuclear energy can be split into a radiation-free element by modern decay processes. If this is not possible until space transport is safe enough to transport nuclear waste, the waste should be disposed of in the sun or another star. By disposing of nuclear waste on alien uninhabited celestial bodies, the cost-intensive research on depletion can be stopped.

Mine water must be pumped out, filtered and detoxified until filter systems underground have absorbed the toxins and then all shafts are filled with filtering soil. If mining has caused damage to the water-impermeable layer of earth, its function must be restored so that poisoning of the freshwater is prevented.

The Institutes of Environmental Health, Occupational Health, Toxics and Hazardous Substances are researching residue-free disposal and how to protect waste disposal and construction workers during demolition, removal and disposal. Special attention is paid to how uncontrolled scattered plastic waste, fine dust and toxins can be collected as effectively as possible and how these substances can be made biodegradable.

6.7 Structural change

Structural change becomes necessary whenever it is recognised that an existing structure of action is harmful to the environment. Certain environmental damage does not become visible in the short term. Often new innovations, such as pesticides or internal combustion engines, have been introduced with good intentions. How nature suffers as a result often only becomes apparent later.

Therefore, the entire population is called upon to observe nature in their surroundings and to report environmental damage in the Environment Directory. The health auditors and physicians do this professionally. The Health Agency collects all reports and connects with all responsible ministries and companies. First of all, the Ministry of Education and its scientists are to clarify whether there is a connection between cause and effect. It is checked whether the cause of the environmental damage is related to the effect described in the report and which influences would still have to be taken into account but are not listed in the report.

The next step is to begin the search for opinions and solutions. Since structural change requires profound changes from many participants, the Minister of Health must convene a committee. Here, decisions are made as to which ministries and companies should be responsible to repair the damage and prevent it in the future.

Structural change may involve interference with economic freedom in order to preserve the health of current and future generations. Structural changes are to be designed in such a way that innovations create added value. These innovations should avoid damage from new technology and thus generate savings or profits at the same time. Only in this way can structural change finance the introduction of reforms and the disposal of inherited burdens without lowering living standards.

6.7.1 Climate change

In today's world, climate change creates the need for structural change and thus sets an example for the procedure for further structural change in the future. The climate change policy of the Ministry of Health is carried out in voting with the other ministries.

The current abrupt climate warming is due to the human emission of carbon dioxide, which was stored by nature in the earth's soil over millions of years of plant growth and has now been released back into the earth's atmosphere by the ton over hundreds of years with exponential growth. The gases carbon dioxide and methane are able to retain heat within the Earth's atmosphere instead of releasing it into space. Deforestation and fallow fields reduce evaporative cooling and alter the global water cycle.

Based on these findings, the Ministry of Health starts its work. Measurements are taken to assess the extent of how fast climate change is progressing and what can stop and reverse it. By evaluating the measures, the time horizon is determined as to how quickly the structural change must be executed in order to have its effect in time.

Structural change ends once global warming has reached the

average temperature of the years 1900 to 1950. Through the acquired knowledge of climate change, humanity can learn how to control the weather without causing damage and how to manage a future naturally induced climate change, for example through a strong volcanic eruption or a coming ice age.

6.7.1.1 Measurements

The necessary data is collected through international cooperation between the research institutions and ministries for environmental affairs. The Ministry of Foreign Affairs supports the Health Agency in negotiating and setting internationally uniform requirements and measures. The Health Agencies in the town halls ensure municipal implementation of the requirements and appropriate measures adapted to the circumstances of each municipality. The people in which the requirements and measures are to be applied must decide on them by majority vote.

The Institute for Toxic and Hazardous Substances singles out pollutants that are responsible for climate change, such as greenhouse gases from fossils, soil layers or farm animals. The health auditors measure who is the originator of such greenhouse gases or clearing and fallowing. In cooperation with the Health Agency, the Company Auditing Agency and its economic auditors determine the costs of the damage caused and the profits made by saving these costs. With the help of the innovation auditors, technical solutions are found that can stop the emission of greenhouse gases as quickly as possible and eliminate past damage. The institutes of the Ministry of Health support the Company Auditing Agency in evaluating the collected data.

6.7.1.2 Measures

Climate change policy consists of preventive measures against the causes of climate change and aftercare measures against the effects of climate change.

As climate change is already showing its effects and causing damage, this damage must be kept to a minimum. The Ministries of Labour and Infrastructure are responsible for the measures they develop in cooperation with the Ministry of Health. All state institutions are accompanied in the implementation by the business consultants of the Company Auditing Agency. All companies can additionally book this service for a fee.

Water scarcity on the one hand and floods on the other are compensated by appropriate structural measures, such as flood basins, dams and dikes.[120] The Ministry of Justice provides the necessary punitive measures for violations through the prosecution of negative externalities and environmental pollution.[121]

The Ministry of Labour is doing its part to prevent the causes of climate change by converting agriculture to permaculture and agri-factories. Water storage and raising the water table is achieved in the short term through bamboo. Soil protection from erosion is provided by perennial cover of any soil area using permaculture.[122] Perennial vegetation at higher altitudes increasingly filters more CO_2 per cubic metre from the air all year round, as well as binding and evaporating more water. The Ministry of Infrastructure ensures the switch from fossil fuels to renewable energy sources that do not produce greenhouse gases and that the originators of structural change bear the costs.[123]

6.7.2 Bioeconomy

The bioeconomy is another structural change triggered by a shortage of raw materials. Regenerative raw materials are replacing fossil raw materials. Through this structural change,

---

120 Ministry of Infrastructure - 8.9.4 Flood Basin, 4.9.1 Water Supply
121 Ministry of Justice - 8.11.6 Negative externalities, 8.6.1 Environmental pollution
122 Ministry of Labour - 19.8.4 Climate change mitigation, 14.3 Environmental protection, 20.7.2.2 Environmental protection assessment, 19.8.7 Nature-based agriculture: Permaculture
123 Ministry of Infrastructure - 4.2 Environmental protection, 8.4 Environmental protection in transport, 9.3 Environmental compatibility

the entire economy is being converted to a circular economy that constantly recycles valuable materials in an inherently stable ecosystem. Products are increasingly produced by genetically programmed growth with a biodegradable nutrient solution than by heating, cooling, moulding and assembling. This structural change ends as soon as all raw materials are renewable or can be completely recycled.

6.7.2.1 Circular economy[124]

The Ministry of Health is responsible for a raw materials policy that ensures resource protection through a circular economy. For this purpose, it examines the use and consumption of raw materials with the Institute of Environmental Medicine and the health auditors and researches their reusability. Based on the data, requirements are made for the production quantities of raw materials that ensure nature's ability to renew itself. Requirements for sectoral product stewardship will regulate the assembly of raw materials into products that ensure their recyclability. The requirements for the recovery of recyclable materials are developed in cooperation with the waste management companies and apply to the manufacturing and processing industries. In addition to recycling, the manufacturing companies also ensure suitable concepts for the avoidance and recycling of waste through their products and their packaging. If it is not possible for companies to dispense with hazardous and non-recyclable waste, they bear the costs of screened and accessible landfill by waste management companies and research into the future avoidance of such waste. Anyone who sells a product must include its disposal costs in the sales price and pay them to the disposal companies. This makes waste disposal free of charge for consumers and public waste bins are widespread. The waste management companies are operated or used by the Ministry of Infrastructure to manage industrial and municipal waste in such a way that it can be fed into the circular economy.[125]

124§189,1 Sustainability: BV Art. 73, §190,6,8 Environmental protection: KV Art.36
125Ministry of Infrastructure - 4.9.2 Waste disposal

The transboundary shipment of waste is only permitted if this is the only way to enable a circular economy. The health auditors monitor compliance with the requirements. The Health Agency is responsible for municipal, continental and international resource efficiency matters when it comes to cooperation with other domestic and foreign authorities.

7 Switching to the new system

The Ministry of Health also takes over the responsibilities of the Ministries of Environment, Nature Conservation and Nuclear Safety. It converts the operation of the Health Agencies to the new requirements. In the process, the Health Agency in the capital city receives instructions from the Minister of Health and, together with the municipal health offices, ensures implementation by persons and companies. The health auditors are pulled together from existing authorities and institutes and incorporated into the Company Auditing Agency. The Ministry of Health cannot fully carry out its work until the responsibility of the regions has been transferred to the national level.

7.1 Digitalisation of health care

The Health Directory is initially an internet-based software on the computers of the persons providing treatment. All health insurance cards are given the functions of the Health Card. The personal patient data is stored on security servers of the Ministry of Health and can only be decrypted in binding with the Health Card. All individual records of treatments are transferred from the physician's computer to the Ministry of Health's server after a visit to the physician and retrieved from there for subsequent treatments by physicians. This eliminates archiving obligations for physicians. The new Medical Fee Schedule replaces the previous rules on fees for physicians and the requirements for minimum health care in the social laws. From then on, billing in the health care system will be exclusively digital.

7.2 Restructuring of the insurance companies

All health insurance companies are transferred to the Free Market Economy and the Ministry of Health establishes its health insurance companies. Long-term care insurance is also transferred to the Free Market Economy. The state long-term care insurance is provided by the General Health Insurance. The distribution of caregivers and care recipients will be operated through the Care Directory in order to provide an intermediary role for caregivers and care recipients. In addition, the need for care and the supply of voluntary and professional helpers can thus be statistically surveyed directly. As soon as there are sufficient contributors to the General Health Insurance care insurance scheme, housing for the disabled will be created in Social Villages under the construction supervision of the Ministry of Infrastructure.

7.3 Conversion of associations, authorities and institutes

The physicians' association takes over the tasks of the existing unifications for physicians.
State institutes for medicines and medical devices are transformed into the Institute for Medicines and Foodstuffs. It becomes part of the health auditors and is their central laboratory. State institutes for vaccines and biomedical medicines also become part of the health auditors and are mainly used for the examination and promotion of research projects as well as the approval of new medicines and current production processes for medical devices.
The state agencies for health education, diseases, poisons and hazardous substances become part of the Institute for Diseases and Vaccines, the Institute for Poisons and Hazardous Substances and the Health Agency and continue their tasks there.

7.4 Use of foundation assets

The state foundations for the environment contribute their foundation assets to the budget of the Ministry of Health. The money is gradually invested in profitable environmental protection projects. First, it is used to finance the establishment of permaculture. As soon as the permaculture growth outstrips the profits of the time, the profits are used to restore the foundation's assets. This is the case after about 5 years. After that, the money is used to finance the energy transition. As soon as energy production is profitable without the addition of raw materials, the profits are used to restore the endowment assets, which should be done after another 10 years. The foundation assets are always spent when environmental damage that has triggered a structural change needs to be remedied.

7.5 Conversion of the old ministries

For the conversion of the old ministries, all departments and units of the old ministries that are changing to this ministry are identified. The organigrams are used to determine whether an entire department and all its units are changing or only individual units. All unsuitable departments and units are dropped. The existing staff adapts its tasks to the new requirements.

Contact form

Dear reader
If you would like to make what you have read come true, in whole or in part, together with other like-minded people, I offer you several possibilities with this contact form. Fill it out, tear out the page and send it by post to:
Andreas Seidl, P.O. Box 1206, 63488 Seligenstadt / Germany

Or send the details to:
Phone: 0049 1522 818 2243 (whatsapp, telegram, signal)
Email: andreas.seidl2022@web.de

Please mark with a cross:
O   I want to found a dynamic People's Party.
O   I want to donate money for implementation.
O   I want contacts with like-minded people in my area.

Forename: _____

Surname: _____

Please fill in only the contact option through which a reply should be made.

Street, house no.:   _____

Postcode, city, country: _____

Phone: _____

Email address: _____